Ambulatory Gynaecology

Withdrawn

Ambulatory Gynaecology

A new concept in the treatment of women

Edited by
Kevin Jones

ISBN 978-1-904752-34-9

Published by the **RCOG Press** at the
Royal College of Obstetricians and Gynaecologists
27 Sussex Place, Regent's Park
London NW1 4RG

Registered Charity No. 213280

RCOG Press Editor: Emma Campbell PhD
Index: Liza Furnival, Medical Indexing Ltd
Design & typesetting: Saxon Graphics Ltd, Derby
Printed in the UK by Henry Ling Ltd, The Dorset Press, Dorchester DT1 1HD

Contents

About the authors

Dr Rupert Broomby FRCA
Specialist Registrar, Anaesthesia
Department of Anaesthetics
Great Western Hospital
Swindon, Wiltshire

Dr Neil Campbell FRCA
Consultant Anaesthetist
Department of Anaesthetics
Great Western Hospital
Swindon, Wiltshire

**Mr Simon A Butler-Manuel MD
MRCOG FRCS(Eng)**
Consultant Gynaecological Oncologist
Department of Gynaecology
Royal Surrey County Hospital
Guildford, Surrey

Mr Theo Giannopoulos MRCOG
Clinical Research Fellow
Gynaecological Oncology
Royal Surrey County Hospital
Guildford, Surrey

Mr Kevin Jones MSc MD MRCOG
Consultant Obstetrician and
Gynaecologist
Department of Obstetrics and
Gynaecology
Great Western Hospital
Swindon, Wilts

Dr Natalia Price MRCOG
Specialist Registrar in Obstetrics and
Gynaecology
John Radcliffe Hospital
Oxford

Mr Simon R Jackson MA MD MRCOG
Consultant Urogynaecologist
John Radcliffe Hospital
Oxford

Mr Valentine Akande PhD MRCOG
Consultant Obstetrician and
Gynaecologist
Southmead Hospital
Bristol

Dr Elinor Medd MB BS MRCOG
Specialist Registrar in Obstetrics and
Gynaecology
Southmead Hospital
Bristol

Mrs C Pearce RGN BA (Hons) MSc
Nurse Consultant, Gynaecology
Department of Obstetrics and
Gynaecology
Great Western Hospital
Swindon
Wiltshire

Miss Zara Haider MRCOG
Clinical Research Fellow
Department of Gynaecology and
Pelvic Ultrasound
St George's Hospital
Tooting, London

Mr Tom Bourne PhD MRCOG
Consultant Gynaecologist
Department of Gynaecology and
Pelvic Ultrasound
St George's Hospital
Tooting, London

Dr Woodruff J Walker FRCR FFR
Consultant Interventional and
Diagnostic Radiologist
Department of Radiology
Royal Surrey County Hospital, and
The London Clinic
Guildford
Surrey

Abbreviations

ACU	assisted conception unit
BMI	body mass index
BSCCP	British Society for Colposcopy and Cervical Pathology
CHAI	Commission for Health Audit and Improvement
CIN	cervical intraepithelial neoplasia
DUB	dysfunctional uterine bleeding
EGU	emergency gynaecology unit
EPU	early pregnancy unit
EWTD	European Working Time Directive
FSH	follicle stimulating hormone
hCG	human chorionic gonadotrophin
HRT	hormone replacement therapy
HyCoSy	hysterosalpingo contrast sonography
LH	luteinising hormone
LLETZ	large loop excision of the transformation zone
MMC	Modernising Medical Careers
MRI	magnetic resonance imaging
NHS	National Health Service
NICE	National Institute for Health and Clinical Excellence
PAF	Performance Assessment Framework
PCOS	polycystic ovary syndrome
RCOG	Royal College of Obstetricians and Gynaecologists
RCT	randomised clinical trial
SHBG	sex hormone binding globulin
THL	transvaginal hydrolaparoscopy
TOT	transobturator tape
TSH	thyroid stimulating hormone
TVT	tension-free vaginal tape
TVUS	transvaginal ultrasound scan

Preface

Ambulatory gynaecology may be an unfamiliar term to many gynaecologists working outside the USA. However, the term is increasingly being adopted in the UK to describe a 'see and treat' management philosophy in outpatient clinics in combination with minimal access surgery in the day surgery unit. In recent years, the Royal College of Obstetricians and Gynaecologists, in collaboration with the British Society for Gynaecological Endoscopy, has run scientific meetings dedicated to 'ambulatory gynaecology'. The adoption of the concept by international and national societies will help promote the management philosophy. This move is timely because a change from traditional care pathways to more cost-effective, patient-centred approaches to medical practice lies at the heart of modern health service management. In light of this we decided to produce a book that sets out how the concept of ambulatory gynaecology can be applied to the main areas of gynaecological practice. I am grateful to the contributing authors who have given their time to write chapters for the book. They are all experts in their fields and they are actively engaged in clinical practice so their contributions are both practical and insightful.

It is hoped that after reading this book the reader will be stimulated to challenge the more traditional models of service delivery in gynaecological practice.

Kevin Jones

1

Introduction

Kevin Jones

Ambulatory gynaecology is a term more commonly used in North America than in the UK. It combines a 'see and treat' management philosophy in outpatient clinics with minimal access surgery in the day surgery unit (Figure 1.1). That is: 'one stop' clinics and 'day surgery' operations replace traditional outpatient consultations and inpatient surgery. Ambulatory gynaecology shortens the care pathway for patients and saves resources (Figure 1.2). Although the term 'ambulatory gynaecology' may be new in the UK, the principle has been applied for some time; for example, in a see-and-treat colposcopy service or an early pregnancy unit.

In order to provide a one-stop service it is necessary to combine the clinical consultation and investigations (Table 1.1) as a single outpatient visit. Minimal access surgery is a vital component of ambulatory gynaecology because it provides an alternative strategy for carrying out common gynaecological operations. The advantages of daycase surgery are extensively documented.

Table 1.1 Specific investigations and treatment for ambulatory gynaecology	
One-stop service	**Investigation/treatment**
Abnormal uterine bleeding	Transvaginal ultrasound scan Endometrial biopsy Hysteroscopy (diagnostic/operative) Office-based endometrial ablation
Colposcopy	Colposcopy Electrosurgical generator/cutting and coagulating attachments (or equivalent laser equipment)
Fertility	Transvaginal ultrasound scan HyCoSy or transvaginal hydrolaparoscopy Hysteroscopy Protocols for medical treatments or referral to ACU
Urogynaecology	Transvaginal ultrasound scan Urodynamic equipment Flexible cystoscopy Office-based continence procedures
Early pregnancy/ emergency gynaecology unit	Transvaginal ultrasound scan Transvaginal ultrasound-guided procedures Serum ßhCG/progesterone Protocols for conservative/medical treatment options

ACU, assisted conception unit; hCG, human chorionic gonadotrophin; HyCoSy, hysterosalpingo contrast sonography

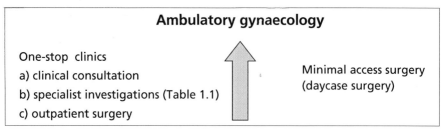

Ambulatory gynaecology

One-stop clinics
a) clinical consultation
b) specialist investigations (Table 1.1)
c) outpatient surgery

Minimal access surgery
(daycase surgery)

Figure 1.1 The components of ambulatory gynaecology

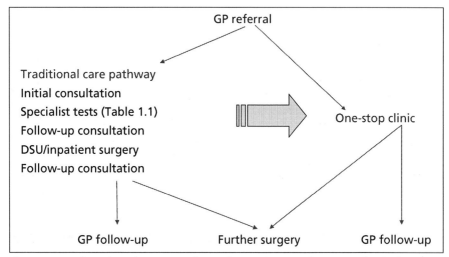

GP referral

Traditional care pathway
Initial consultation
Specialist tests (Table 1.1)
Follow-up consultation
DSU/inpatient surgery
Follow-up consultation

One-stop clinic

GP follow-up   Further surgery   GP follow-up

Figure 1.2 Changing the care pathway for patients with gynaecological conditions; DSU, day surgery unit; GP, general practitioner

To deliver an ambulatory gynaecology service, gynaecologists will have to work closely with primary care doctors. They will need to develop protocols and referral guidelines so that the management in primary care is not duplicated in the hospital environment and patients are directed to the correct multidisciplinary teams (Figure 1.3). They will also have to learn new skills and professional bodies are introducing training courses and standards for accreditation which are facilitating this (see Appendix 1.1: Useful websites). Gynaecologists will also have to accept different ways of working, where they are part of a multidisciplinary team providing organisational continuity rather than the traditional model of a lone consultant skilled in every aspect of obstetrics and gynaecology providing personal patronage.[1]

This book is not intended to be used as a 'step by step' manual of how to set up and run an ambulatory gynaecology service, although it is hoped that there is enough practical detail to facilitate this process. Neither is it intended to provide an extensive review of the literature, although key references and useful websites are cited. The book has been written with the intention of describing how national guidelines, such as those produced by the Royal College of Obstetricians and

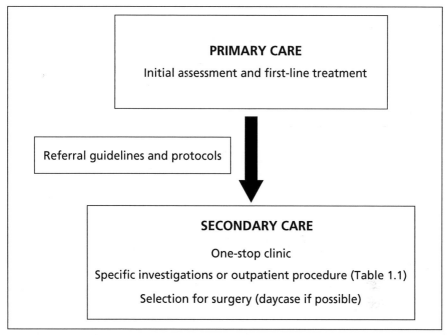

Figure 1.3 Integration of primary and secondary care to deliver an ambulatory gynaecology service

Gynaecologists (RCOG) and other national bodies, can be integrated into modern gynaecological practice in the context of the Government's National Health Service (NHS) plan.

The overall objectives of ambulatory gynaecology

A large number of gynaecological conditions can now be dealt with efficiently on an outpatient basis. Wherever possible, this involves one visit (one stop). In this way, repeat visits for investigations can be avoided, as may hospital admissions. In some instances it is possible to offer medical management of conditions previously treated surgically. If surgery is required, the aim is to use a minimal access approach in the day surgery unit. By adopting modern advances in surgical technology and challenging traditional gynaecological practice, clinical services can be redesigned for the benefit of women. These new approaches to gynaecology can be delivered more cost effectively than the management strategies previously provided, which is in keeping with the NHS delivery plan.[2,3] The overall objectives of an ambulatory gynaecology management philosophy are to:

- shorten the whole treatment process (care pathway) for women
- speed up recovery and return to work for women
- increase outpatient procedures

- increase daycase rates
- free up capacity on inpatient theatre lists and hospital wards
- reduce the number of elective operations cancelled by the hospital
- reduce the overall unit cost of treatment
- deliver the principles of governance and controls assurance.

The strategic context

Primary care trusts in the UK now pay hospitals through an incentive system using a standard tariff, based on national human resources group benchmarks. Work will therefore need to be undertaken locally to drive unit costs closer to the UK average. Hospitals are to be inspected by the Commission for Health Audit and Improvement (CHAI) and will continue to be allocated a star rating based on performance against an increasing range of Performance Assessment Framework (PAF) indicators. CHAI will be given new powers to implement special measures if NHS trusts do not perform at the expected level. The star rating of a trust currently affects its ability to access the NHS Performance Fund but in the future it will also affect the size of the trust's baseline allocation.

There are currently no PAF indicators directly relating to gynaecology. However, gynaecology activity affects the overall bed and theatre pool of the hospital and as a result has a direct impact on a range of key performance indicators, including trolley waits and surgical access times. The adoption of an ambulatory gynaecological management philosophy whenever possible will help individual NHS trusts to achieve these objectives. Not only does this benefit individual women, it also benefits all the patients using the hospital service because it makes economic sense.

The strategic vision set out in the NHS Plan[2,3] provides the context for the development of ambulatory gynaecological services and is summarised in the following five components:

1. Providing a balanced range of services that promote health and wellbeing and tackle health inequalities.
2. Ensuring safe and high-quality care with an increasing element of choice (the right care).
3. Fast and convenient (at the right time).
4. As close to the home as possible (in the right place).
5. Ending delays at all stages in the elective and emergency system.

The NHS Plan[2,3] sets out the key targets that will need to be achieved to deliver the vision. In particular, ambulatory gynaecology will help to reduce waiting times by increasing overall capacity for the hospital, reducing bed occupancy and contributing to the infrastructure needed for services to be redesigned around the patients. Hospitals are now expected to deliver an 18-week patient pathway from GP referral to the start of treatment by the end of 2008 for all patients (www.18weeks.nhs.uk). The whole care pathway is captured in the 18-week time frame from referral through to treatment, including all tests and outpatient consultations up to the start of treatment. For ambulatory gynaecology patients, the target is a minimum of 90% of admitted pathways (daycase) and 95% of non-admitted (outpatients) pathways will be completed in less than 18 weeks. To achieve this, the first outpatient appointment will occur within 4 weeks of referral (by direct booking), if daycase surgery is required this will occur within 14 weeks of the oupatient consultation. The care pathway is set out in Figure 1.4. The numbers in the flow diagram relate to the key set out in Table 1.2. Ambulatory gynaecology is a management strategy which is ideally suited to meeting these

Table 1.2 Care pathway key

18-week clock status code		18-week clock reason		
Stop 18-week clock at this appointment	30	First Definitive Treatment		Patient has been given 1st treatment/medication to treat condition at this appointment
	34	Decision not to treat		It is decided that no treatment is required
	35	Patient Declined Offer of Treatment		Patient has decided that they do not want treatment
	32	To start Period of Active Monitoring (consultant initiated)		Clinician has decided that patient should be managed by watchful waiting
	31	To start Period of Active Monitoring (patient initiated)		Patient has decided that they should be managed by watchful waiting
	33	ADULT patient has **DNA 1st appointment**		Adult patient has not arrived for first appointment
Continue 18-week clock as still awaiting treatment	10	**CHILD** patient has **DNA 1st appointment**		Child patient has not arrived for first appointment; clock continues to tick
	20	Patient still awaiting first treatment		Patient is still awaiting first treatment for condition and clock continues
Continue 18-week clock already stapped	90	Patient has previously had 1st treatment		Patient has previously had first treatment for condition and continues to recieve care
	91	Patient is still being Actively Monitored/ Watchful Waiting		Patient is in period of watchful waiting for this condition and continues to be so
Start new 18-week clock	11	Decision to treat after returning from Period of Active Monitoring		Start new 18-week clock as patient returns from watchful waiting

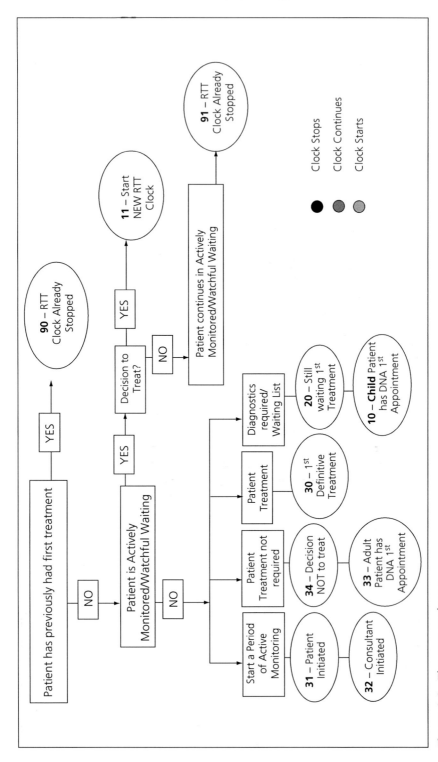

Figure 1.4   The care pathway

targets. Furthermore the NHS Plan calls for the development and implementation of new and innovative ideas to help reshape and improve services, particularly those that increase capacity and day case rates.

Service delivery and training

Initiatives such as Modernising Medical Careers (MMC), the 'Hospital at Night' project, the European Working Time Directive (EWTD) and the new 'time sensitive' contract for consultants (Table 1.3) will have a profound influence on the way hospital doctors are trained and work together in the future. These initiatives are integral parts of the Government's strategy for reforming the health service,[4,5] which will be combined with a significant increase in consultant numbers.

Until recently, consultants in the UK have been required to be expert in all aspects of the specialty and junior doctors were principally used for service provision. This is the basis of a consultant-led rather than a consultant-provided service. The Government's reforms of the NHS and the EWTD[6,7] are rapidly changing this traditional model of training and healthcare provision.[8] They are providing the right environment to redesign clinical services based on one-stop management and minimal access (daycase) surgery which are the components of an ambulatory gynaecology service.

As a consequence of these reforms, trainees were being awarded a Certificate of Completion of Specialist Training with less clinical experience than their predecessors. In future, they will be awarded a more general Certificate of Completion of Training. The drive to acquire a smaller number of selected special interest skills and to focus job descriptions on areas of subspecialism will lead to a wide disparity in clinical ability between individuals, who will have a narrower focus of expertise. The challenge for the profession is how to restructure our units in a way that implements these reforms and uses the new breed of specialist for the patient's benefit. The fundamental change that would have to occur to achieve this is to redefine the working relationship between consultants, who would no longer act as the head of a 'firm' in isolation from their colleagues. The establishment of multidisciplinary services would facilitate this. It would also enable the

Table 1.3 UK government reforms of the NHS	
Reform	**Consequence**
Modernising Medical Careers	Shifting training towards a competency-based, shorter training system
The European Working Time Directive, time-sensitive consultant contract	Juniors and consultants will work shorter hours
The Hospital at Night project	Change the way all clinical staff work in hospitals in the out of hours period
Increasing consultant numbers	Not enough middle grades to maintain the traditional 'firm' structure

NHS to move towards a consultant 'provided' service where patients are the responsibility of the department, not an individual doctor. Under this system, patients are managed according to the unit's protocols and not a particular consultant's preference.

Establishing an ambulatory gynaecology service

To make these changes successful, a number of changes need to occur.

Minimal access surgery training

Minimal access surgery will need to be taught to all trainees. Surgeons should be able to perform operative as well as diagnostic endoscopic procedures, so that a see-and-treat procedure is offered to patients. This will help to reduce the number of inpatient procedures because more operations will be performed as day cases. It will also help to reduce repetition of operative procedures under general anaesthesia because diagnosis and treatment can occur at the same time.

Ultrasound scanning by the gynaecologist

In the UK, the majority of gynaecology consultations involve referring the woman for an ultrasound scan. It is a pivotal investigation in gynaecological practice and a recurring theme throughout this book. Ultrasound scanning by the gynaecologist could become a routine part of the consultation rather than being delegated to radiographers in a separate department on a separate day after a period on a waiting list.

The RCOG and British Society for Gynaecological Endoscopy are establishing special skills modules and subspecialist training programmes to facilitate training and to regulate accreditation in minimal access surgery and transvaginal ultrasound (Appendix 1.1).

Generic referral

Referral to hospital by general practitioners is moving towards a system of referrals where 'generic' patients are the responsibility of the whole department, not an individual consultant. Under this system, individual patients are looked after by multidisciplinary teams with an appropriate special interest working together on a common clinical problem.[5,6] Management strategies are evidence based and protocol driven. This helps to achieve uniformity of practice and equality of patient care.

Approved protocols and guidelines

In order to adopt a generic referral system, evidence-based, NICE-approved protocols and referral guidelines must be in place for general practitioners to follow.

This will ensure that management in primary care is not duplicated in the hospital environment and that women are directed to the correct multidisciplinary teams (Figure 1.3).

Monitoring, audit and patient safety

If accredited specialists (consultants) worked together in the operating theatre or the clinic, it would provide everyone with the opportunity to monitor each other's performance, update techniques and expand repertoires, and reciprocate teaching opportunities. The arrangement would facilitate the acquisition of new clinical skills in order to deliver an ambulatory gynaecology service. It would also facilitate audit, patient safety and uniformity of management.[9] The main argument put forward for maintaining the traditional system usually focuses on continuity of patient care as a result of personal patronage of individual patients. Where a multidisciplinary team approach has been adopted as part of an ambulatory gynaecology service, this is often replaced by organisational (system) continuity.[10–12]

Auditing the service and patient satisfaction surveys

Participation in clinical audit is a mandatory requirement for all doctors working in the modern health service. It is a key component of clinical governance and contributes to an individual NHS trust's Clinical Negligence System for Trusts status, which has important financial implications that in turn affect clinical services. Several organisations including the RCOG produce guidelines on a range of topics that are relevant to ambulatory gynaecology. These guidelines contain suggested topics for audit. They can be used as audit standards to measure performance and to answer the question: 'are we doing what we are supposed to be doing?'. The audit cycle (Figure 1.5) should form part of any clinical service and establishes the principle of clinical quality assurance. In the more established areas of ambulatory gynaecology, such as the colposcopy service, there are

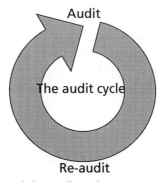

Audit

The audit cycle

Re-audit

Figure 1.5 Clinical audit and the audit cycle

national audit standards that need to be met (Chapter 3) with respect to establishing and running a service.

The concept of patient satisfaction is also important in the modern NHS. At the level of the individual clinician this may be used as part of the appraisal process. At the level of an organisation providing innovative and new services it is vital to demonstrate that the needs of the local community are being met.

Summary

Ambulatory gynaecology combines one-stop see-and-treat clinics with day surgery. There are core skills that must be applied and new working practices adopted to deliver the service. The authors have described the application of a one-stop, see-and-treat management philosophy combined with minimal access surgery to their area of specialist expertise, emphasising the benefits compared with traditional work practices.

References

1. Jones KD. Gynaecological training in a consultant delivered service: a European perspective. *The Obstetrician & Gynaecologist* 2005;7:126–8.
2. Department of Health. *A First Class Service: Quality in the NHS*. London: The Stationery Office; 1998.
3. Department of Health. *The NHS Plan. A Plan for Investment, A Plan for Reform*. London: The Stationery Office, 2000.
4. Wanless D. *Securing Our Future Health: Taking a Long-term View, Final Report*. London: The Stationery Office; 2002.
5. Pickersgill T. The European working time directive for doctors in training. *BMJ* 2001;323:1266–5.
6. Burke D. Making the European Working time Directive a reality. *BMJ* 2002;324: s66–7.
7. Lissauer R. The future workforce. *BMJ* 2002;324:s73–4.
8. British Medical Association Health Policy and Economic Research Unit. *The Future Healthcare Workforce*. London: BMA, 2002.
9. Charlton R. Continuing professional development (CPD) and training. *BMJ* 2001;323:2–3.
10. Freer SD. Whither continuity of care? *N Engl J Med* 1999;341:850–2.
11. Manian FA. Whither continuity of care? *N Engl J Med* 1999;340:1362–3.
12. Krogstad U, Hofoss D, Hjortdahl P. Continuity of hospital care: beyond the question of personal contact. *BMJ* 2002;324:36–8.

Appendix 1.1

Useful websites

Association of Early Pregnancy Units: www.earlypregnancy.org.uk

British Society for Colposcopy and Cervical Pathology: www.bsccp.org.uk

British Society for Gynaecological Endoscopy: www.bsge.net

NHS Cancer Screening Programmes: www.cancerscreening.nhs.uk

Ectopic Pregnancy Trust: www.ectopic.org

General Medical Council: www.gmc-uk.org

Human Fertilisation and Embryology Authority: www.hfea.gov.uk

International Continence Society: www.icsoffice.org; http://www.ukcs.uk.net

International Pelvic Pain Society: www.pelvicpain.org.uk

Miscarriage Association: www.miscarriageassociation.org.uk

National Health Service. Delivering the 18 week patient pathway:
www.18weeks.nhs.uk

National Institute for Health and Clinical Excellence: www.nice.org.uk

Royal College of Obstetricians and Gynaecologists: www.rcog.org.uk

Scottish Intercollegiate Guidelines Network: www.sign.ac.uk

2

Anaesthesia and analgesia for outpatient gynaecology

Rupert Broomby and Neil Campbell

Introduction

The intention of this chapter is to provide advice for the anaesthetic care of women undergoing outpatient gynaecological surgery. The purpose of anaesthesia is to allow a woman to undergo surgery in safety and comfort, with as little disturbance as possible of normal daily activities. Although general anaesthesia is certainly possible in an office or day unit environment, it requires extra investment in personnel, equipment and facilities, and necessitates extra preoperative preparation and postoperative recovery. Accordingly, it should be reserved for situations where local anaesthesia is impractical or is likely to be inadequate. A similar argument holds for spinal or epidural anaesthesia. The long latency and recovery times associated with epidural anaesthesia make it impractical for rapid turnover day surgery, where the aim is to efficiently treat multiple patients in a surgical session. Spinal anaesthesia allows for a more rapid turnover; but for 'office' type day cases, problems remain with delayed postoperative mobilisation, sphincter control and spinal headache. We will, however, consider the use of only local anaesthetic techniques, with or without sedation.[1]

Sedation can facilitate many simple daycase gynaecological procedures, allowing a comfortable, stress-free operation with early mobilisation and discharge. In this chapter, we will look at a definition of safe sedation; the staff, equipment and drugs needed to achieve this; and aspects of patient selection and postoperative analgesia.

Conscious sedation is described as 'a technique in which the use of drug or drugs produces a state of depression of the nervous system enabling treatment to be carried out, but during which verbal contact with the patient is maintained throughout the period of sedation'.[2] The drugs and techniques used should carry a margin of safety wide enough to render loss of consciousness unlikely. Sedation techniques have the potential, however, to cause life-threatening complications, which can be minimised by following guidelines on the use of sedation. Formal written protocols should be available for each department that uses sedation techniques.

Sedation techniques should be undertaken only in appropriately equipped premises. Staff administering sedative drugs should receive training in the technique. Sufficient support staff should be available to deal with any emergency and to provide proper supervision during the recovery stage. Written protocols should be available and systems in place to ensure compliance. Women should be appropriately selected and informed of available options for pain relief.[1,3]

Patient selection

Patient selection should be based on social and medical factors.

Social factors

- Women must be willing to undergo the procedure under sedation
- There should be a responsible adult available to care for the woman for the first 24 hours after discharge
- Patients' homes should be suitable for postoperative care with access to bathroom, toilet and kitchen facilities, and use of a telephone.[4]

Medical factors

- The woman should be fully fit or any chronic disease should be controlled[4,5]
- Ahead of any procedure, risk factors should be identified, which may be done using a simple questionnaire (Appendix 2.1), taking into account the proposed procedure. Identification of risk factors initiates any need for further investigations.

Obesity

- Obesity carries risk the of associated diseases such as diabetes, ischaemic heart disease, cerebrovascular disease and hypertension.
- Additional factors, such as patient positioning, moving and anatomical problems, may make intravenous access and regional anaesthesia difficult.
- The obese airway may be difficult to manage.

Obesity is defined by body mass index (BMI) of more than 30 kg/m². A BMI of more than 35 kg/m² is considered morbidly obese. Patients with a BMI of more than 30 kg/m² show increased sensitivity to sedation. There is also an increased incidence of sleep apnoea in the morbidly obese category. It is therefore advisable to avoid sedation in the morbidly obese and show caution in patients with a BMI of more than 30 kg/m².[6]

Staffing

It is preferable for a second qualified member of staff to provide sedation and monitoring of the woman throughout the procedure.[3] Nevertheless, in the UK, most often a single operator administers the sedation and performs the procedure. This practice has become acceptable for minor procedures when a single drug such as midazolam is used. Midazolam has a large safety margin, making airway obstruction or significant respiratory depression unlikely in the fit patient. If the operator is unable to maintain close proximity to the airway or if other, more potent drugs are used, a second member of staff should be available to monitor the woman. More potent drugs include intravenous opioids or short acting anaesthetic agents such as propofol.[1]

It has been suggested that staff should have skills equivalent to 2 years' training in anaesthesia and they must hold a current Advanced Life Support Provider certificate.[3] At this level of training it may be difficult to provide adequate numbers of staff to provide a service. There is as yet no formal qualification in the UK for 'sedationists', but development of training courses should be encouraged. The minimum standard of care acceptable is to designate a trained member of the nursing staff to monitor the patient, if the only medically qualified member of the team is both giving the sedation and performing the procedure. Staff should also be available to safely nurse the woman through the recovery period. Emergency procedure protocols should be devised and practised.

Equipment

Patient trolleys should be capable of being tipped head down, to prevent aspiration of gastric contents, if gastric reflux occurs while protective reflexes are impaired. Appropriate resuscitation equipment should be immediately available and staff made familiar with its use. Examples of suitable emergency equipment are given in Box 2.1 and Figure 2.1.[3]

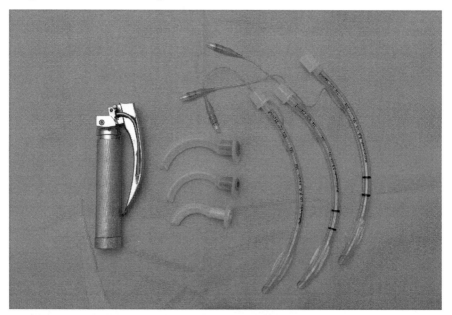

Figure 2.1 Laryngoscope, Guedel airways and endotracheal tubes

---

Box 2.1 Emergency equipment

Airway equipment:
Self-inflating resuscitation bag with oxygen reservoir and tubing (Ambu® bag [Ambu International A/S, Glostrup, Denmark])
Backup oxygen supply (cylinder)
Oxygen tubing with mask
Pocket face mask
Guedel oropharyngeal airways
Clear face masks sizes 3, 4 and 5
Laryngoscopes with long and short blades
Cuffed oral endotracheal airway
Gum elastic bougie
Scissors and ribbon gauze
Laryngeal mask airway sizes 3 and 4 (if trained in their use)
Suction apparatus including suction catheters and Yankauer suckers

Intravenous administration equipment:
Venous cannulae sizes 20 gauge to 14 gauge (standard wire gauge)
Intravenous fluid and blood administration set
Intravenous fluids (crystalloid and colloid)
Various syringes and needles
Adhesive dressings
Antiseptic skin wipes
Tourniquet

Monitoring:
Cardiac defibrillator with cardiac monitor and appropriate connection devices
Defibrillation gel pads
Noninvasive automatic blood pressure monitor
Pulse oximeter
Sphygmomanometer
Stethoscope

Monitoring

Basic monitoring during outpatient gynaecological procedures should include pulse oximetry, noninvasive blood pressure and electrocardiogram monitoring. Pulse oximetry is mandatory in all cases of sedation. Blood pressure and electrocardiogram monitoring may not be essential in young, healthy individuals, but should always be considered in elderly women, especially if there are cardiovascular problems (Figure 2.2).[1,3]

Oxygen must be available. Devices for delivery may include nasal or facial masks (Figure 2.3a–c). There should also be a means of delivering positive pressure oxygen. There should always be a backup supply of cylinder oxygen.

Resuscitation equipment should be available, staff should be familiar with its use and there should be a programme for regular checking and maintenance. This equipment should include basic airway devices, intubation equipment, self-inflating bags for ventilation (Ambu® bags, Figure 2.4), emergency drugs, including any antidotes to drugs used for sedation, and a cardiac monitor and defibrillator (Figure 2.5).

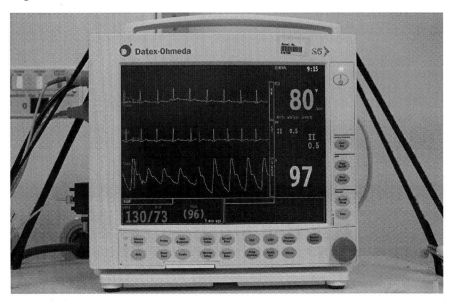

Figure 2.2 Monitor showing blood pressure, electrocardiogram and pulse oximetry measurements

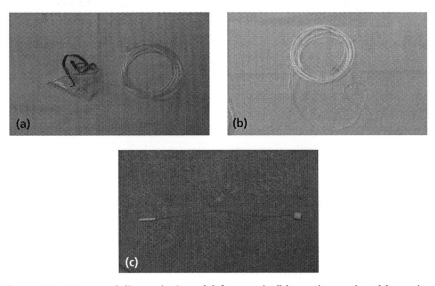

Figure 2.3 Oxygen delivery devices: **(a)** facemask, **(b)** nasal speculae, **(c)** nasal sponge

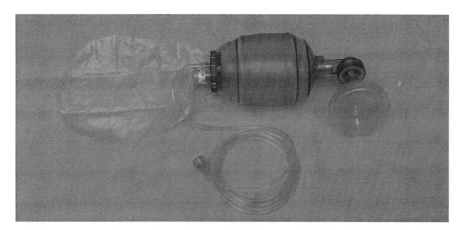

Figure 2.4   Self-inflating resuscitation bag with oxygen reservoir and tubing (Ambu® bag)

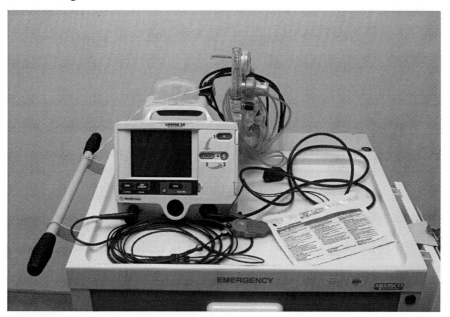

Figure 2.5   Cardiac monitor and defibrillator

Administration

Drugs may be given by the oral, intravenous or inhalation routes. The aim is to prevent or treat pain and anxiety associated with the surgical procedure.

Anxiety can also be reduced using simple behavioural techniques to reassure the woman during the time prior to the procedure. A careful explanation and time spent with the woman to answer questions and ameliorate concerns will often achieve this.

If using intravenous sedation, secure intravenous access is mandatory and oxygen must be given with pulse oximetry monitoring. Oxygen may given by facemask or by nasal delivery, using appropriate equipment.[1]

The choice of drugs should address the need for both analgesia and sedation. Oral analgesics are best used in combination with a single intravenous agent such as midazolam. Avoiding combinations of intravenous drugs can avoid the complications of crossing from sedation to anaesthesia. Knowledge of the pharmacodynamics and pharmacokinetics of the available agents will allow anticipation of potential complications. Some of the common drugs and their pharmacological features are discussed below.

The sedationist should always check that the appropriate equipment is available and working before starting the procedure. During administration of sedation the woman should never be left alone. A record should be kept of the sedation technique used. Documentation should include observations of vital signs during the procedure, as well as drugs given and relevant information from preoperative questioning.

Recovery and discharge

Patients should remain in a designated recovery area until fully awake, orientated and comfortable. Prior to discharge, the operator should review patients. They should receive information about what to expect in the first 24 hours, and should have a supply of appropriate analgesics.

It is advised that patients avoid alcohol, cooking and operating machinery until the following day. Following sedation, it is advised to avoid driving for 24 hours.[4]

Commonly used drugs

Midazolam

Midazolam is a benzodiazepine frequently used to sedate patients during minor procedures. Like all benzodiazepines it causes anxiolysis and hypnosis, and has anticonvulsant activity. It also has the beneficial effect of causing anterograde amnesia, so patients often have no recall of mild discomfort occurring during the procedure, following administration.[7]

It is presented as a clear solution with a pH of 3.5. At this pH it is a water-soluble molecule, but at physiological pH it forms a different structure, which makes it more lipid soluble. Lipid solubility allows the molecule to cross lipid membranes, thus giving a faster onset of action. It may be given orally, intramuscularly or intravenously. When midazolam is used for intravenous sedation, the dose should be titrated in boluses of 0.5–2 mg. Effects are usually seen within 90 seconds. Women who are elderly or unwell may be sensitive to the effects so the dose should be reduced accordingly.

This drug is metabolised in the liver and inactive metabolites are excreted in the urine. The half-life is between 1 and 4 hours.

Other effects include cardiovascular depression with associated hypotension, and respiratory depression, especially when combined with intravenous opioids. Pulse oximetry monitoring and oxygen therapy should always be used.

Midazolam has a generous therapeutic window, which allows its safe use as a sedative, but a large dose (0.3 g/kg) can induce anaesthesia. It should be remembered that it is not a good analgesic agent and its use to control pain may result in overdose. Pain is better controlled by analgesics or local anaesthetics.

Paracetamol

The adult dose of paracetamol is 1 g given 4–6 hourly, (maximum 4 g per day). It can be given orally or rectally. The mechanism of action is not fully understood but it is thought to have a central effect that inhibits prostaglandin synthesis. Paracetamol is a good, simple analgesic with few adverse effects.

Nonsteroidal anti-inflammatory drugs

Diclofenac

This drug is available as intramuscular, oral and rectal preparations. It is useful for mild-to-moderate postoperative pain. The adult dose is 50–100 mg given 8 hourly to a maximum dose of 150 mg in 24 hours.

Ibuprofen

Available as tablets or paediatric elixir, this drug has the lowest incidence of adverse effects of all the nonsteroidal anti-inflammatory drugs. The adult dose is 200–400 mg, 8 hourly.

Opioids

Opioids have a variety of effects, which are brought about by action at opioid receptors. Although the opioids all have similar effects, there are substantial differences in the pharmacokinetics and pharmacodynamics of the different drugs. As well as their analgesic effect, opioids may cause many adverse effects, some of which are listed in Box 2.2.

Box 2.2 Adverse effects of opioids
Respiratory depression
Mild bradycardia and hypotension
Nausea and vomiting
Central nervous system effects of sedation, euphoria and dysphoria
Constipation
Pruritus
Miosis
Urinary retention

Tolerance and dependence can occur over time. Most of the serious adverse effects are dose dependent and are not problematic when using the less potent preparations usually given for mild to moderate analgesia.

Codeine
This drug is a commonly used oral opioid. A dose of 30–60 mg is given 4–6 hourly. Common adverse effects are nausea, vomiting and constipation.

Dihydrocodeine
This is a similar drug with similar potency and adverse effects to those of codeine. A dose of 30 mg is given 4–6 hourly. Combination analgesics are also available, many of which combine paracetamol 500 mg with various amounts of codeine or dihydrocodeine.

Antiemetics

Postoperative nausea and vomiting may be less likely following sedation than after general anaesthesia, but can still occur. Antiemetics commonly used include antihistamines (e.g. cyclizine, prochlorperazine), dopamine antagonists (e.g. metoclopramide, domperidone), 5-hydroxytryptamine 3 antagonists (ondansetron) and steroids (e.g. dexamethasone). Acupuncture at the P6 point has also been shown to have an antiemetic effect.

Local anaesthesia

Local anaesthetics function by blocking sodium channels to prevent conduction of nerve action potentials. They can be used in three ways to produce pain relief during or after a procedure:

1. To block a specific nerve or group of nerves.
2. As local infiltration around the site of the surgery.
3. For topical administration.

Local anaesthetics cause reversible blockade of action potentials in autonomic, sensory and motor nerve fibres. The drug binds to sodium channels from within the axon membrane, preventing sodium influx and a subsequent action potential. Features of the block are affected by drug characteristics, site of injection, concentration and dose, and use of additives.

Drug characteristics
Local anaesthetics are poorly water-soluble, weak bases that are mainly highly protein bound. They may be classified as esters or amides, depending on the nature of linkage between aromatic and amine parts of the drug. Properties of commonly used local anaesthetic agents are summarised in Table 2.1 and complications of their use are described in Box 2.3.

Box 2.3 Complications of local anaesthetics

Toxic dose:

From either systemic absorption or accidental intravascular injection.

Overdose may cause central nervous system and, subsequently, cardiac symptoms.

As the plasma concentration rises, the woman may experience peri-oral tingling, light-headedness, visual disturbances, confusion and tremors, and may become restless. Further rises in toxic dose cause grand mal seizures, coma and respiratory arrest.

The effect of local anaesthetics on cardiac muscle causes slowing and prolongation of PR and QRS intervals, allowing re-entry arrhythmias and ventricular fibrillation. Cardiac toxicity typically occurs at seven times the dose needed to produce central nervous system toxicity for lidocaine, and at four times the dose for bupivacaine.

Recommended safe maximum doses for local anaesthetic agents are given in Table 2.1. Local anaesthetics are typically formulated as a percentage concentration – for example, lidocaine is normally presented as 0.5%, 1% or 2% strength. One millilitre of 1% will contain 10 mg of the drug.

The treatment of toxicity owing to local anaesthetics centres on basic resuscitation and symptomatic relief.

Recognition is important, followed by the Airway, Breathing, Circulation resuscitation protocol. Adequate tissue oxygenation will prevent permanent damage. Anticonvulsants may be given if necessary (typically benzodiazepines diazepam or midazolam intravenously). Further use of local anaesthetics should be avoided until plasma levels are certain to be safe.

Systemic effects of vasoconstrictors:

Adrenaline may cause tachycardia, agitation, pallor and arrhythmias. Effects are usually short-lived.

Neurological damage and neurotoxicity:

Great care should be taken to avoid intraneural injection. Neuropathies may also occur from poor positioning in theatre during prolonged procedures.

Methaemoglobinaemia:

A complication specific to prilocaine in doses above 600 mg in adults, caused by oxidation of the iron atom in haem to the ferric (Fe^{3+}) state. Causes dark skin appearance, which may be appear similar to cyanosis. Pulse oximetry readings may be inaccurate. Usually reverts spontaneously. If symptomatic (headaches and/or dyspnoea), it can be treated with a reducing agent such as methylene blue.

Allergy to local anaesthetics:

Allergies are rare and are more likely to occur with esters than with amides. Amide local anaesthetics can be safely used for women with genuine allergy to ester local anaesthetics. Some preservatives mixed with local anaesthetics may also cause allergic reactions.

Infection and haematoma formation:

Haematomas can be caused by injection at any site but usually cause only minor effects. Infection risk can be reduced by the use of sterile techniques, skin preparation and sterile equipment.

Table 2.1 Properties of commonly used local anaesthetics				
Agent	pKa	Protein binding (%)	Concentration (%) needed for equivalent potency among all agents	Recommended safe maximum dose (mg/kg)
Esters				
Amethocaine	8.5	76	0.25	1.5
Cocaine	8.7	n/a	1.0	3.0
Amides				
Lidocaine	7.9	64	1.0	3.0 (7.0 with adrenaline)
Bupivacaine	8.1	96	0.25	2.0
Ropivacaine	8.1	94	1.0	3.5
Prilocaine	7.9	55	1.0	6.0

The pKa value determines the onset of action (the higher the pKa the slower the onset of action). Protein binding determines the duration of action (the greater the protein binding the longer the duration of action.) n/a = data not available

Vasoconstrictors such as epinephrine (adrenaline) or felypressin may be added to reduce absorption and prolong the duration of action. Addition of a vasoconstrictor is particularly useful with lidocaine, which causes more vasodilatation than most other local anaesthetics. Cocaine causes vasoconstriction without the use of additives.

Topical anaesthesia

Local anaesthetic creams such as EMLA® (eutectic mixture of local anaesthetic; AstraZeneca, Luton, Beds) and tetracaine (amethocaine) are particularly effective for the reduction of pain from venepuncture. EMLA® is a combination of prilocaine 2.5% and lidocaine 2.5%.

Topical anaesthesia has been used for minor gynaecological procedures. EMLA® has been shown to provide good pain relief for procedures involving surface tissues, such as the removal of genital warts and hysteroscopy.[8] It can also be used to reduce the pain of local anaesthetic injection for deeper tissues.

Complications following sedation
Inappropriate administration of sedatives

It has become apparent that in the past sedation techniques involved doses of sedatives that produced effects closer to general anaesthesia than to conscious sedation. In the event of loss of verbal contact, the woman should receive care equivalent to that given with a general anaesthetic. Good patient assessment and a good understanding of the procedure will allow correct judgement of drug doses and appropriate determination of the need for analgesia. Sedative medications like benzodiazepines have poor analgesic properties. Use of these agents without adequate analgesia will more than likely result in overdosage. Good analgesia can be achieved either by analgesic medication taken with the sedatives, or by the use of local anaesthesia.

Excessive doses of benzodiazepine may be reversed with flumazenil, which is a competitive antagonist for benzodiazepines. Flumazenil also has some inverse agonist properties, which can cause agitation, anxiety, nausea, vomiting and seizures. Careful consideration should be given before it is used. Its relatively short half-life means its effects may wear off before those of the benzodiazepines.

The effects of opioids may be reversed using naloxone but note that it has a shorter half-life than some of the drugs it may be used to reverse.

Regurgitation

Relaxation of the lower oesophageal sphincter can cause regurgitation of stomach contents. Patients should be starved prior to sedation, similarly to general anaesthesia. Adequate starvation times are 6 hours for solid food and 2 hours for clear fluids.

Vasovagal episodes

These episodes may cause hypotension and bradycardia, and can cause dizziness and collapse. Symptomatic bradycardia should be treated with an anticholinergic medication such as atropine.

Inadequate analgesia

As well as postoperative pain and anxiety, inadequate analgesia may lead to unnecessarily large doses of sedation during the procedure.

Anaphylaxis

Anaphylactic reactions are rare but potentially fatal. Between 1995 and 2001 there were, on average, 319 cases per year of anaphylactic reactions reported to the Medicines and Healthcare products Regulatory Agency, with a 3.7% fatality rate.[9] Of all these cases of anaphylaxis, 55 per year were related to general anaesthesia and the fatality rate was 10%. Of the agents related to anaesthesia, neuromuscular blocking drugs are the most frequent cause of anaphylaxis (62%). The evidence also shows a gender difference, with females two and a half times more likely to suffer a reaction than males. Other agents that were implicated in anaphylaxis were latex (17%), antibiotics (8%), hypnotics (5%), colloids (3%) and opioids (3%).

When performing sedation with intravenous medication, it is therefore important to be able to recognise and treat anaphylactic reactions. Presenting features

Box 2.4 Treatment for suspected anaphylaxis[9] (from *Suspected anaphylactic reactions associated with anaesthesia*. AAGBI, 2003, with permission)

Management of a patient with suspected anaphylaxis during anaesthesia: model operating procedure/guideline:

1. Stop administration of all agents likely to have caused the anaphylaxis.
2. Call for help.
3. Maintain airway, give 100% oxygen and lie patient flat with legs elevated.
4. Give adrenaline (epinephrine). This may be given intramuscularly in a dose of 0.5–1.0 mg (0.5–1.0 ml of 1:1000) and may be repeated every 10 minutes according to the arterial pressure and pulse until improvement occurs.

Alternatively, 50–100 micrograms intravenously (0.5–1.0 ml of 1:10 000) over 1 minute has been recommended for hypotension with titration of further doses as required.

Never give undiluted epinephrine 1:1000 intravenously.

In a patient with cardiovascular collapse, 0.5–1.0 mg (5–10 ml of 1:10 000) may be required intravenously in divided doses by titration. This should be given at a rate of 0.1 mg/minute stopping when a response has been obtained.

Paediatric doses of epinephrine depend on the age of the child. Intramuscular epinephrine 1:1000 should be administered as follows:

> 12 years 500 micrograms IM (0.5 ml)
6–12 years 250 micrograms IM (0.25 ml)
> 6 months – 6 years 120 micrograms IM (0.12 ml)
< 6 months 50 micrograms IM (0.05 ml).

Start rapid intravenous infusion with colloids or crystalloids. Adult patients may require 2–4 litres of crystalloid.

Secondary therapy:

1. Give antihistamines (chlorpheniramine 10–20 mg by slow intravenous infusion).
2. Give corticosteroids (100–500 mg hydrocortisone slowly IV).
3. Bronchodilators may be required for persistent bronchospasm.

may be cardiovascular collapse, bronchospasm, cutaneous features (rash, urticaria and erythema), generalised oedema, pulmonary oedema or gastrointestinal symptoms. The wide variety of presenting features can make initial diagnosis difficult. It must be suspected and treated promptly in sudden cases of cardiovascular collapse or severe bronchospasm. An example of a treatment regimen, as used for anaesthesia, is shown in Box 2.4.

References

1. Wildsmith JAW. *Implementing and ensuring safe sedation practice for healthcare procedures in adults*. London: UK Academy of Medical Royal Colleges and their Faculties; 2001.
2. Skelly AM. Analgesia and sedation. In: Watkinson A, Adam A, editors. *Interventional radiology*. Oxford: Radcliffe Medical Press; 1996. p. 3–11.

3. Department of Health. *Conscious sedation in termination of pregnancy. Report of the Department of Health Expert Group.* London: 2002.
4. Association of Anaesthetists of Great Britain and Ireland. *Day surgery.* London: AAGBI; 2005.
5. Proudfoot J. Analgesia, anaesthesia, and conscious sedation. *Emerg Med Clin North Am* 1995;13:357–79.
6. De Jong RH. Body mass index: risk predictor for cosmetic day surgery. *Plast Reconstr Surg* 2001:108;556–61; discussion 562–3.
7. Nadin G, Coulthard P. Memory and midazolam conscious sedation. *Brh Dent J* 1997;183:399–407.
8. Zilbert A. Topical anaesthesia for minor gynaecological procedures: a review. *Obstet Gynecol Surv* 2002;57:171–8.
9. Association of Anaesthetists of Great Britain and Ireland. *Suspected Anaphylactic Reactions Associated with Anaesthesia.* London: AAGBI; 2003.

Appendix 2.1

Sample questionnaire used to determine risk factors before surgery (with permission from the University Hospital of North Staffordshire NHS Trust)

Social Factors

Will You?

Be able to be driven home by private car... YES/NO

Have someone to take you home... YES/NO

Have a telephone at home... YES/NO

Have easy access to a lavatory... YES/NO

Have some one at home to look after you for 24 hours... YES/NO

Medical Factors

Have You Suffered From Any Of The Following:

Heart Attack... YES/NO

If so, when?... _____

Angina... YES/NO

Shortness of Breath... YES/NO

   If *YES*, answer the following:

      Do you feel breathless:

         At rest... YES/NO

         On lying flat... YES/NO

         On exertion... YES/NO

         On climbing stairs... YES/NO

      How far can you walk before becoming breathless?.. _____

Asthma... YES/NO

Bronchitis... YES/NO

High Blood Pressure... YES/NO

Heart Murmur... YES/NO

Rheumatic Fever... YES/NO

Convulsions or Fits... YES/NO

Kidney or Urinary trouble... YES/NO

Anaemia or other blood problems... YES/NO

Excessive bleeding or bruising... YES/NO

Hepatitis... YES/NO

Severe indigestion or heartburn... YES/NO

Diabetes... YES/NO

      If YES, Is it controlled by diet... YES/NO

                Tablets... YES/NO

                Insulin... YES/NO

Arthritis... YES/NO

Muscle disease (e.g. muscular dystrophy) or weakness... YES/NO

Deep vein thrombosis or blood clot in lungs (PE)... YES/NO

Swollen ankles... YES/NO

Do you have a pace maker?... YES/NO

Do You have sickle cell disease or trait?... YES/NO

Please give your:

Height...   Weight...

Blood pressure...   Heart rate...

   (Measured by nursing staff)

Do you have any allergies?

Do you take any regular medicines?   Please List

Do you smoke?

Please list any previous operations

Did you have any surgical or anaesthetic complications?

3

Colposcopy services

Theo Giannopoulos and Simon Butler-Manuel

Introduction

Colposcopy is probably the first example of a one-stop gynaecology service where the concept of a see-and-treat management philosophy was introduced successfully.

The colposcope was invented in 1925, by Hans Hinselman, and colposcopy was initially developed separately from cervical cytology. The introduction of acetic acid (1938) and the Pap test (1940) helped to develop colposcopy as a reliable diagnostic test, complementary to cytological screening. Owing to the invention, in 1989, of large loop excision of the transformation zone (LLETZ), which can be used in the outpatients setting, few situations still necessitate treatment under general anaesthesia.

In the UK, cervical cytology is used as a primary screening test and colposcopy as a secondary tool (Figure 3.1). The NHS cervical screening programme was introduced in 1988 and is now acknowledged as a notable story of success, saving around 1,300 lives per year.[1]

National targets: national service frameworks, guidelines and consensus documents

The British Society for Colposcopy and Cervical Pathology (BSCCP) and the Royal College of Obstetricians and Gynaecologists (RCOG) have produced guidelines for the provision of colposcopy services in the UK.[2,3]

These guidelines emphasise the value of training, audit and team work and set standards of care. Previous standards that relate to quality in the colposcopy clinic, such as staffing, privacy and changing facilities, have been made more stringent. The views of women are also taken into account. All these changes may have resource implications but this is unavoidable if healthcare is to be quality driven.

An important goal is to ensure that the colposcopy service becomes more focused on women with substantial abnormalities. Women who are at very low risk of developing cervical cancer should not undergo colposcopy or at the very least should be returned to community surveillance as quickly as possible. This practice not only is an efficient use of resources but also recognises the possible negative health impact of unnecessary colposcopy in women who have a very

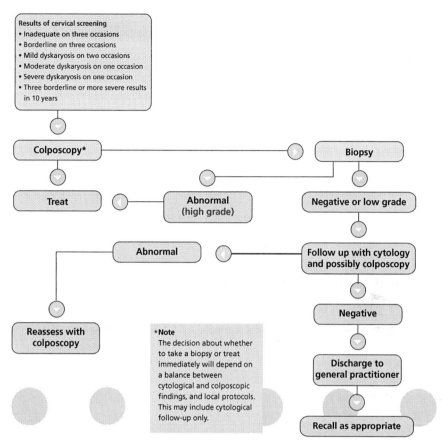

Figure 3.1 Protocol for management of abnormal results of cervical screening

low risk of developing cervical cancer. In fact, there is evidence that many women suffer significant anxiety from receiving an invitation for colposcopy and this anxiety can compromise compliance with subsequent screening and follow-up.[4]

The recent major change in the core of the cervical screening programme is the recommendation for referral after one mildly dyskaryotic sample. This change will increase the workload in the short term. A rapid return to community-based cytology surveillance is also recommended, however, for all women who have normal colposcopy examination results and low-grade abnormalities. Women who are at low risk will be returned to routine recall more quickly, whereas those at high risk will be maintained on follow-up for up to 10 years after treatment. In addition, the widespread use of liquid-based cytology smears is expected to reduce the number of referrals of consecutive inadequate or borderline smears. Taken together, it is judged that this strategy offers both safety and eventually efficiency.

The RCOG has published a list of standards, established by consensus (Box 3.1). It is acknowledged that few clinics will be able to achieve all of these

Box 3.1 Main points of the RCOG guidelines

- The colposcopy service should have a designated lead clinician and lead nurse
- All colposcopy should be performed by trained and accredited colposcopists or by trainees under supervision
- Clinics should record the waiting times for both new patients and treatments
- All clinics should adhere to local written protocols, which should reflect published national guidelines and should ensure adequate data collection for quality assurance and annual review
- The service should aim to minimize intervention in women who do not have cervical intraepithelial neoplasia
- Participation in audit and continuing medical education is mandatory.

standards, but good progress has been made toward achieving these goals and this progress must continue and be encouraged.

Organisation of the service: infrastructure required, clinic set up, staff, training and equipment

We have now moved away from the concept of a 'clinic' to one of a 'quality-assured service'. This is a far more comprehensive concept because it broadens the focus to include all aspects of the diagnostic, therapeutic and surveillance activity and does not concentrate purely on clinic-based activity.

Colposcopy should be organised as a quality-assured service, whatever the setting, and should be run by a team using protocols based on guidelines. Any problems arising in connection with practice should be addressed in a confidential and supportive manner. Leadership, organisation, informatics and training should all be considered part of such a service.

A hospital-based programme coordinator or lead colposcopist should:

- be ideally at consultant level
- make a major time commitment to fulfil this role
- lead the service and specialist team
- devise appropriate written protocols
- ensure that quality-assurance targets are monitored
- ensure that multidisciplinary meetings, including histopathology and cyto-pathology staff, are held at least twice per year
- ensure accreditation of the team through the BSCCP/RCOG
- comply with the re-certification process every 3 years
- ensure that continuing professional development is pursued by all team members.

There must be at least two nurses for each colposcopy clinic.

The primary nurse should:

- be trained in counselling

- be the named nurse dedicated to the unit
- not have other concurrent outpatient duties
- provide support to the patient.

A second nurse:

- assists in the preparation between patients for cervical sampling and treatment
- does not need to be a fully trained nurse.

Adequate clerical and secretarial support is required:

- for timely communication with patients and the general practitioner
- for data collection
- to ensure effective, failsafe mechanisms.

The clinic's facilities should protect the woman's dignity. They must include a private area with changing facilities, toilet facilities and a permanently sited room used specifically for colposcopy. Refreshments must be available and there must be separate waiting and recovery areas.

The number of visitors to the unit should be limited, but women should be allowed to have a friend or relative present if they wish. In addition, the woman's permission should be sought prior to colposcopy if any additional staff, who are not essential for performance of the procedure, are present. The resources required to set up a colposcopy clinic are set out in Box 3.2.

Box 3.2 The equipment required to set up a colposcopy clinic

A permanent couch with stirrups and colposcope

Appropriate sterilisation facilities

Guidelines for laser or diathermy equipment

Emergency guidelines

Trained staff

Adequate resuscitation equipment

Software to facilitate collection of data

Television monitoring facilities for patients who wish to watch the procedure

A colposcopy tray containing:
- A bivalve speculum and an endocervical speculum
- Cotton wool and cotton-tip swabs
- Sponge-holding forceps
- Biopsy forceps
- Three small galley pots containing normal saline
- Acetic acid and Lugol's iodine (iodine–potassium iodide solution)
- Thin Prep Pap test and cervical broom for taking a cervical smear
- A variety of electrosurgical diathermy ball and loop electrodes
- Electrosurgical generator.

Box 3.3 Main cytological abnormalities that require referrals

Mild dyskaryosis (but it remains acceptable to recommend a repeat smear)

Moderate or severe dyskaryosis

Three consecutive inadequate or borderline samples

Borderline nuclear change in endocervical cells

Mild dyskaryosis or worse after previous treatment for cervical intraepithelial neoplasia

Possible invasion

Glandular neoplasia.

Clinical indications and referral guidelines for general practitioners and hospital specialists

Most of the referral guidelines are based on professional consensus. Local or regional factors may, however, have a strong influence on practice.

The main cytological abnormalities that require referrals (in accordance with the 2004 BSCCP guidelines) are shown in Box 3.3.

The key change is the recommendation for colposcopy after one dyskaryotic smear. Women with a mild dyskaryotic result should be seen and assessed but not necessarily treated. To prevent possible over-treatment, they should not be managed in a see-and-treat scenario.

The recommendation for women with moderate or severe dyskaryosis remains unchanged because this group can have up to 90% risk of high-grade cervical intraepithelial neoplasia (CIN). Consecutive inadequate samples may be produced from a background of invasive cancer in the presence of an inflammatory process, and there may be bleeding on contact.

Women with consecutive borderline smears are at increased risk of development of high-grade CIN over time. Borderline glandular cells are associated with high rates of preinvasive (17–40%) and malignant (4–16%) disease.[2,3]

Management protocols

Management must be seen to help enhance the efficiency and efficacy of the service.

In particular, clinics that provide a see-and-treat policy must ensure that women who are offered treatment at their first visit are sent adequate and appropriate information in advance of their appointment.

At least 90% of women with a test result of moderate or severe dyskaryosis should be seen in a clinic within 4 weeks of referral. For mild abnormalities, this time can be up to 8 weeks.

All these principles, although primarily designed for NHS practice, may be extended to the private sector in the UK.

Practical techniques

All women who need treatment must have a colposcopic assessment and their consent must be recorded. There is no obviously superior conservative surgical technique for the treatment and eradication of CIN.[5] Ablative techniques are suitable, however, only when the entire transformation zone is visualised, there is no evidence of glandular abnormality or invasive disease and there is no major discrepancy between cytology and histology results.

Treatment should be performed with adequate local analgesia (Chapter 2). A mixture of local anaesthetic (lignocaine) and local vasoconstrictor (octapressin) is used to infiltrate the cervix to the point that the tissues are seen to blanch. The infiltration should be around and not inside the transformation zone because theoretically malignant cells can be introduced in the stroma, and the technique is effective in around 2 minutes.

In some cases, general anaesthesia should be offered but the reasons should be documented in the colposcopy record. This proportion of women should not exceed 20%.

Most colposcopy clinics in the UK use LLETZ as an excision method. There is evidence, however, that needle excision of the transformation zone or straight wire excision of the transformation zone are more likely to produce clear margins because they can remove a large lesion in a single piece.[6] They have the potential to eliminate the need for cold knife biopsy under general anaesthesia.

LLETZ is a simple, cheap technique, which is easy to teach and can usually be performed in less than 10 minutes. Good exposure of the cervix is necessary. In multiparous women, the lateral vaginal walls protrude occasionally through the speculum blades and cause obstruction. In these cases, a condom can be wrapped around the speculum to keep the vaginal walls away from the cervix. There is also a specially designed, four-bladed speculum that can be used for this purpose. A choice of loops is available for LLETZ.

Good haemostasis is achieved if the loop is moved slowly but additional haemostatic measures are occasionally needed (usually coagulation with diathermy or by application of Monsel's solution). There must, however, be fewer than 5% of cases of primary haemorrhage that require a haemostatic technique in addition to the treatment method applied.

When excision is used, at least 80% of specimens should be removed as a single sample. Removal of the transformation zone in multiple fragments can increase the difficulties encountered in histopathological assessment. More importantly, if microinvasive disease is present, it may be impossible to allocate a substage or define completeness of excision. For ectocervical lesions, excisional techniques should remove tissue to a depth of greater than 7 mm.

Cryocautery and cold coagulation should be used for only low-grade CIN as they have a poor rate of clearance of CIN3 (high-grade CIN). They are, however, very good for treatment of secondary bleeding after LLETZ.[7] Laser ablation requires expensive equipment but a laser excisional cone can give a single histology specimen.

All treatments must be recorded. The proportion of patients admitted as inpatients owing to treatment complications must be fewer than 2%.

Accreditation and training

In the UK, colposcopy is carried out predominantly as part of the NHS Cervical Screening Programme. In this context, colposcopy should be performed by only BSCCP certified colposcopists or trainee colposcopists under supervision.[7]

There is a structured training programme that leads to the award of the RCOG/ BSCCP Certificate in Colposcopy (Diagnostic or 'D'). An optional treatment module leads to the award of the RCOG/BSCCP Certificate in Colposcopy (Therapeutic or 'T'). The diagnostic training programme involves:

- Direct supervision of 50 colposcopy cases (of which at least 20 must be new cases, of which ten must be high-grade disease)
- Indirect supervision of 100 cases (of which at least 30 must be new cases, of which 15 must be high-grade disease)
- Completion of the log book
- Presentation of ten clinical commentaries
- Histopathological and cytopathological sessions.

The average duration of training is 18 months. Entry requirements for the programme are membership of the BSCCP,[8] recognised nursing or medical qualification and attendance at a BSCCP accredited Basic Colposcopy Course.

Conclusions

Colposcopy is the first example and the trend setter of the one-stop gynaecology clinic.

The concept of a quality-assured service has now evolved and includes all aspects of diagnostic, therapeutic and surveillance activity. The realisation of quality-assured colposcopy through the NHS Cervical Screening Programme in the UK has been a considerable achievement with proven success.

References

1. NHS Cancer Screening Programmes [www.cancerscreening.nhs.uk].
2. Luesley DM, Leeson SC, editors. *Colposcopy and programme management: guidelines for the NHS Cervical Screening Programme.* NHSCSP Publication No. 20. Sheffield: NHS Cancer Screening Programme; 2004.
3. Prendiville W, Walker P, Jordan J, Shafi MI. *Standards for service provision in colposcopy services.* London: Royal College of Obstetricians and Gynaecologists, 2006.

4. Marteau TM, Kidd J, Cuddeford L. Reducing anxiety in women referred for colposcopy using an information booklet. *Br J Health Psychol* 1996;1:181–9.
5. Martin-Hirsch PL, Paraskevaidis E, Kitchener H. Surgery for cervical intraepithelial neoplasia. *Cochrane Database Syst Rev* 1999;(3):CD001318.
6. Panoskaltsis T, Ind TE, Perryman K, Dina R, Abrahams Y, Soutter WP. Needle versus loop diathermy excision of the transformation zone for the treatment of cervical intraepithelial neoplasia: a randomised controlled trial. *BJOG* 2004;111:748–53.
7. Ostergard DR. Cryosurgical treatment of cervical intraepithelial neoplasia. *Obstet Gynecol* 1980;56:231–3.
8. British Society for Colposcopy and Cervical Pathology [www.bsccp.org.uk].

4

Abnormal uterine bleeding

Kevin Jones

Introduction

The aim of a one-stop service for abnormal uterine bleeding – menorrhagia and postmenopausal bleeding – is to provide rapid access, ultrasound-based clinics for women, where a see-and-treat management philosophy is provided.

This approach allows abnormal uterine bleeding to be dealt with efficiently, on an outpatient basis, often with just one visit. Repeat visits for consultations and investigations can thus be avoided, as may hospital admissions. The aim is to supply a diagnostic and management plan at the same visit. For almost all women, this involves undergoing a transvaginal ultrasound scan (TVUS). Some may need an endometrial biopsy, or an outpatient hysteroscopy. The use of saline hydrosonography may also be helpful. If further treatment is required, women can be offered medical therapy with a progestogen-containing intrauterine system (Mirena®, Schering Health Care Ltd, Burgess Hill, UK). With the development of second-generation devices, endometrial ablation can be performed in the out-patient setting in selected patients. If outpatient treatment is not possible, women can be treated in the day surgery unit. Women with malignant disease can be fast-tracked to the oncology multidisciplinary team for treatment.

Epidemiology, guidelines and national targets

Menorrhagia

In the UK, 5% of women of reproductive age present to their family doctor annually seeking help for menorrhagia.[1] The majority of women have no underlying pathology detected on investigation by the gynaecologist. In such circumstances, women are diagnosed as having dysfunctional uterine bleeding (DUB). The RCOG reports that 42% of the 90 000 hysterectomies performed each year in the UK are for DUB.[2] Rare systemic causes of excess menstrual bleeding such as abnormal thyroid function and haematological diseases can be excluded with appropriate blood tests. The most common organic intrauterine causes of menorrhagia can be excluded with ultrasound scanning and hysteroscopic examination with tissue sampling.

In 1999, the RCOG developed guidelines for the treatment of menorrhagia.[3,4] The guidelines stated that all women with menorrhagia should be offered medical therapy, and/or the Mirena® intrauterine contraceptive device, in the community before referral to hospital (Box 4.1). Some traditional prescribing practices were shown to be unhelpful and the advice was that they should be discontinued (Box 4.2). The guidelines set out the indications for referral to hospital after a failed trial of medical therapy (Figure 4.1). The second-line management of women with menorrhagia is best carried out in a one-stop clinic (Figure 4.2), and this was also set out in the RCOG's national guidelines.[4] Second-line medication can be offered in the hospital setting (Box 4.3); otherwise, if the woman has completed her family and wishes to avoid a hysterectomy, she should be offered an endometrial ablation procedure (Box 4.4). Although the RCOG was the first national body to set out guidelines for the management of heavy menstrual bleeding, the National Institute for Health and Clinical Excellence has subsequently published an algo-rithm for managing this condition (Figure 4.3).[5] The NICE guidelines do not differ significantly from the original RCOG guidelines.

Box 4.1 RCOG recommendations for the initial management of menorrhagia

In women with a history of heavy cyclical menstrual blood loss over several consecutive cycles without any intermenstrual or postcoital bleeding:

- An abdominal and pelvic examination should always be performed
- A full blood count should always be obtained
- Tranexamic acid and mefenamic acid are effective treatments for reducing heavy menstrual blood loss
- Combined oral contraceptives can be used to reduce menstrual blood loss
- A progestogen-releasing intrauterine device (Mirena® intrauterine contraceptive device) is an effective treatment
- Long-acting progestogens, which render most women amenorrhoeic with continued use could be considered.

Box 4.2 Unhelpful practices for the management of menorrhagia

- Thyroid function tests do not need to be routinely performed in the initial evaluation of menorrhagia unless the woman has symptoms or signs of hypothyroidism
- No other endocrine investigations are necessary in the investigation of menorrhagia
- An endometrial biopsy is not required in the initial assessment of menorrhagia
- Low-dose, luteal-phase administration of norethisterone is not an effective treatment for menorrhagia
- Etamsylate, at currently recommended doses, is not an effective treatment for menorrhagia.

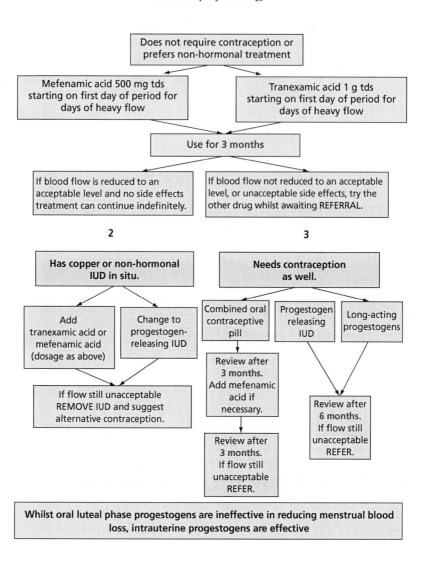

Figure 4.1 The initial management of menorrhagia: when to refer to hospital

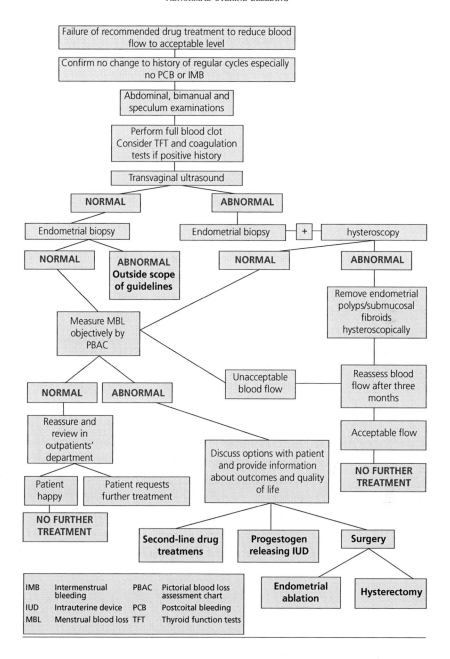

Figure 4.2 The secondary management of menorrhagia

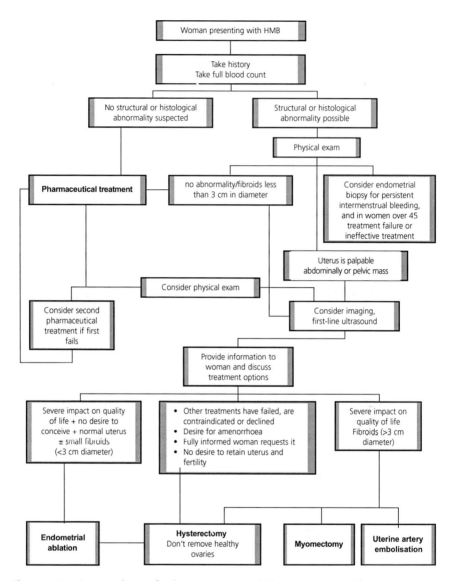

Figure 4.3   Care pathway for heavy menstrual bleeding(HMB) (from NICE guideline)[5]

Box 4.3 Second-line drug treatments for menorrhagia[4]

Danazol, gestrinone, and gonadotrophin-releasing hormone analogues
- are effective in reducing heavy menstrual loss
- have side effects that limit their long-term use.

A progestogen-releasing intrauterine device
- is an effective treatment for menorrhagia
- should be considered as an alternative to surgical treatment
- can be offered to women in the community.

Box 4.4 Surgical treatments for menorrhagia[4]

- A dilatation and curettage is not therapeutic in cases of heavy menstrual bleeding
- If intrauterine pathology such as submucous fibroids or polyps are found during ultrasonic or hysteroscopic investigation, these should be removed hysteroscopically
- Endometrial ablative procedures are effective in treating menorrhagia
- Hysterectomy is an established, effective treatment for menorrhagia
- The widespread use of hysterectomy as a treatment for menorrhagia should be balanced against its potential mortality and morbidity.

Postmenopausal bleeding

This finding represents a common clinical problem in primary care, largely owing to suspicion of an underlying endometrial malignancy. Consultations with general practitioners for postmenopausal bleeding are most frequent in women aged 50–59 years, at 14.3 per 1000 population during 1999–2000.[6] The absolute risk of endometrial cancer in non-users of hormone replacement therapy (HRT) who present with postmenopausal bleeding ranges from 5.7% to 11.5%.[7,8] From a symptomatic perspective, postmenopausal bleeding describes the occurrence of vaginal bleeding 12 months or more after the last period. By contrast, unscheduled bleeding is the term used for breakthrough bleeding occurring in women on cyclical HRT or any bleeding in women taking tibolone (Livial®, Organon, Cambridge, UK) or continuous combined HRT (Box 4.5).

Box 4.5 Unscheduled bleeding or breakthrough bleeding in women on HRT

For sequential regimens, abnormal bleeding may:
- be heavy or prolonged at the end of the progestogen phase, or
- occur at any time (breakthrough bleeding).

For continuous combined regimens, abnormal bleeding may:
- occur after the first 6 months of treatment, or
- occur after amenorrhoea has been established.

> **Box 4.6** Cut-off levels for endometrial thickness on TVUS in women with postmenopausal bleeding or unscheduled bleeding in women using HRT
>
> An endometrial thickness of 3 mm or less:
> - is seen in women who have never used HRT
> - is seen in women who have not used any form of HRT for ≥ 1 year
> - is seen in women who are using continuous combined HRT
> - indicates that no further action need be taken
> - requires further investigations if symptoms recur.
>
> An endometrial thickness of 5 mm or less:
> - is seen in women on sequential combined HRT presenting with unscheduled bleeding.

The Scottish Intercollegiate Guidelines Network has produced evidence-based guidelines for the investigation of postmenopausal bleeding.[6] The guidelines state that the risk of endometrial cancer is high enough to recommend referral for investigation of all non-HRT users who experience postmenopausal bleeding, and all women who use HRT and experience abnormal bleeding. A flow chart on the investigation of women with postmenopausal bleeding can be downloaded from the Scottish Intercollegiate Guidelines Network website.[6] The second-line management of women with postmenopausal bleeding is best carried out in a one-stop clinic, in conjunction with a multidisciplinary oncology team. The consultation should take place within a time frame determined by national guidelines (within 2 weeks of referral by the general practitioner in the UK) because of the suspicion of malignancy (Figure 4.4). The guidelines also recommend that TVUS is the primary diagnostic test of choice (Box 4.6), and this test should be supported by hysteroscopy and endometrial biopsy where necessary.[6]

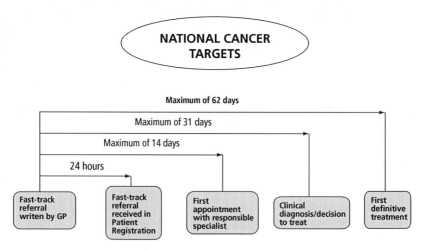

Figure 4.4 UK national targets for the management of patients with a potential diagnosis of cancer

Organisation of the service

The one-stop clinic

One-stop, see-and-treat clinics for the management of abnormal uterine bleeding are becoming increasingly common in UK hospitals, but the correct primary diagnostic tool remains undecided.[9] Some gynaecologists favour TVUS, whereas others rely on hysteroscopy. What is agreed is that multiple hospital visits and inpatient hysteroscopy and curettage under general anaesthesia are no longer considered acceptable strategies for the management of abnormal uterine bleeding.[3,4] The patient care pathway is changing, increasingly, to outpatient-based management strategies in order to avoid this situation. These one-stop clinics offer a combination of TVUS, rigid or flexible hysteroscopy, with directed or blind endometrial biopsies. The change in management philosophy together with advances in technology now allow diagnostic as well as operative procedures to be performed in the outpatient setting.

In order to establish and run a one-stop service for abnormal uterine bleeding, a large, comfortable and private clinical area to carry out consultations and examinations is required. There should also be, ideally, a separate area for patients to get changed, and to be recovered in. A team of dedicated nursing staff who are familiar with the equipment and have an empathy with patients is vital to the running of a successful clinic. A 'vocal local' is often more useful than a local anaesthetic, and a skilled communicator can frequently prevent a vasovagal episode. A fan and a separate chair, positioned so that the accompanying person can to sit close to the patient's head, are helpful in this respect as well. An examination couch with a fold-down section and stirrups are mandatory for achieving easy access to the pelvic organs. We find it helpful to have sterile 'family planning' packs prepared. These packs contain the most commonly used instruments, such as a Cusco speculum, a tenaculum, sponge forceps, dilators, a dental syringe, a fluid receiver, and swabs. It is also advisable to have available a range of different sized speculums, suturing equipment and silver nitrate sticks. There should also be easy access to resuscitation equipment, including oxygen, and the staff working in the clinic should be appropriately trained to use this equipment.

The success of a service depends on the ability to collate the various results from the investigations and then communicate effectively and quickly to the patient and general practitioner. It should also be possible for the service to be audited, which requires dedicated secretarial support and, if possible, a database. A number of commercial database systems exist for the storage of data, including digital images. These systems allow a written report to be generated immediately for the referring physician and patient, and they facilitate audit and research.

Transvaginal ultrasound scan

The development of TVUS has enabled the gynaecologist to obtain high-resolution images of the uterus and ovaries. This has facilitated the accurate diagnosis of intra-cavity focal pathology, such as submucous fibroids and endometrial polyps.

Endometrial cancers, endometrial hyperplasia, adenomyosis and, rarely, estrogen-producing ovarian tumours can also be detected. This is achieved with high-frequency (6–7.5 MHz) transducers located inside probes, which can be placed in close proximity to the pelvic organs. Abdominal probes are used to visualise pelvic masses that extend beyond the focal length of the vaginal probe (approximately 10 cm). The use of saline hydrosonography further enhances the views of the endometrial cavity and endometrium by acting as a negative contrast agent. Colour flow Doppler imaging can provide additional information about blood flow and vascularity but it does not have a role in the routine assessment of abnormal uterine bleeding.

Hysteroscopy

Individual gynaecologists have preferences for rigid, flexible, or disposable hysteroscopy systems. There is also variation in the use of saline solution or carbon dioxide as a distension medium. There is a wide range of products on the market, made by a number of different instrument companies.

Carbon dioxide distension using an insufflator with an automatic pressure control is the gaseous distension medium of choice. The insufflation system should be able to keep the pressure at 100–120 mmHg at a flow rate of 30–60 ml/min (corresponding to a uterine pressure of 40–80 mmHg). The advantage of carbon dioxide gas is that it does not distort the view of the intrauterine cavity, and it does not spill onto the patient or surgeon. It permits an extremely detailed evaluation of the endometrial physiology. In theory, it is possible to perform minor surgery using carbon dioxide, although a liquid medium is preferable for surgical hysteroscopy.

Low-molecular-weight liquid media can be either electrolyte or non-electrolyte solutions. Electrolyte solutions include 5% and 10% dextrose, 4% and 6% dextran, and saline or physiological solutions, which are frequently used to distend the uterine cavity in cases in which no electricity is applied. The advantages of low-molecular-weight liquid media are widespread availability, low operating costs and physiological absorption. Their disadvantages are that they are fairly miscible with the blood and require constant perfusion of the liquid to maintain cavity distension. They also spill during and after the examination. The system used to control pressure flow can be a gravity flow system, in which a bag is raised to a height of 90–100 cm above the patient. This height is sufficient to achieve a pressure of approximately 17 mmHg, which causes the liquid to flow down the outer sheath of the hysteroscope by the force of gravity. Pressure cuff devices similar to a sphygmomanometer may also be inflated around the bag exerting pressure on it. Irrigation is achieved either by passive backflow out through the cervix or by connecting the hysteroscope outflow connector to an electronic suction and irrigation pump.

Light sources are particularly important and high-quality light sources such as xenon give the best results. In general, a power of 17 watts is sufficient for routine interventions. For special interventions or when miniature telescopes are used, 30 watts are recommended. The camera system is also extremely important and there are many companies who produce high-quality equipment for this purpose.

It is necessary to have a good hysteroscope, which can be either flexible, rigid or a partially disposable system. Rigid telescopes are available with different directions of view: 0 degrees, 12 degrees and 30 degrees. Normally, the 30-degree telescope is used for diagnosis. Hysteroscopes of different diameters are available. Miniaturised endoscopes (2 mm telescopes) are generally used for diagnostic hysteroscopy, whereas a small outpatient telescope with a diameter of 2.9 mm can be used for diagnostic and operative hysteroscopy. A single-flow operating sheath of 4.3 mm diameter or continuous-flow outer sheath tubes of 5 mm diameter may be used and sheaths with operating channels are available.

The technique used to perform a diagnostic hysteroscopy is crucial for a successful examination. The woman should be placed in the dorsolithotomy position with her legs in stirrups. The perineum is cleaned thoroughly with cotton wool soaked in antiseptic or physiological solution. A 10 ml bolus of local anaesthetic may be injected into the anterior lip of the cervix using a dental syringe. Alternatively a four-quadrant block of the cervix may be administered. The light source, distension medium and camera are connected to the hysteroscope, which is then inserted into the cervical canal under direct vision. A panoramic view of the uterine cavity should be obtained and both ostia visualised. Any areas of suspicious endometrium should be examined and, if necessary, additional instruments can be inserted down the operating channel of the hysteroscope to perform directed biopsies or minor surgical procedures.

Following the procedure, it is important to sterilise the instruments in conjunction with the central operating room sterilisation department and the responsible member of staff should be adequately trained to do this.

Results: evidence-based medicine

Endometrial sampling and hysteroscopy

For many years, the most widely used technique for obtaining a sample of endometrium for histological evaluation was dilatation and curettage; however, this procedure has numerous limitations. The false negative rate of dilatation and curettage is between 2% and 6% for the diagnosis of endometrial cancer and hyperplasia.[10,11] Such figures also hold true for obtaining an endometrial sample by other methods, such as the Pipelle® endometrial sampler (Laboratoire CCD, Paris, France).[12] These problems arise owing to sampling errors. Stock and Kanbour[11] demonstrated this point by performing dilatation and curettage immediately prior to hysterectomy in 50 women. They showed that in 30 of the 50 women (60%), less than half of the cavity was sampled. More recently, the evaluation of endometrial pathology

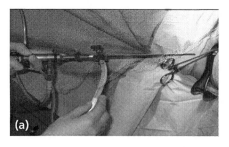
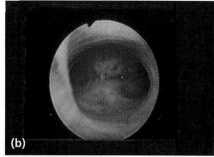
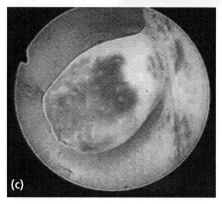

Figure 4.5 **(a)** Hysteroscopy, with views of **(b)** an atrophic uterine cavity and **(c)** an endometrial polyp

with direct vision has become possible with hysteroscopy (Figure 4.5). This procedure allows for directed biopsies to be taken, thereby minimising the theoretical risk of sampling errors. If the hysteroscope has no operating channel with which to take biopsies, however, sampling is still in effect 'blind'. The literature suggests, nevertheless, that hysteroscopy provides an increase in diagnostic information. Gimpelson and Rappold[13] studied 276 patients who underwent both hysteroscopy and dilatation and curettage. Hysteroscopy yielded more information in 44 patients while dilatation and curettage gave more accurate information in only 9 patients. The use of hysteroscopy seems to offer particular advantages for the diagnosis of endometrial polyps and submucous myomas.

Transvaginal ultrasound scan

The endometrium

TVUS is a highly sensitive method for the detection of endometrial abnormalities.[14,15] In the assessment of postmenopausal bleeding, the finding of a regular endometrial echo with a thickness of less than 5 mm (Figure 4.6) has been shown to have a high negative predictive value for the presence of pathology.[16] The premenopausal endometrium is, however, a dynamic structure and when other

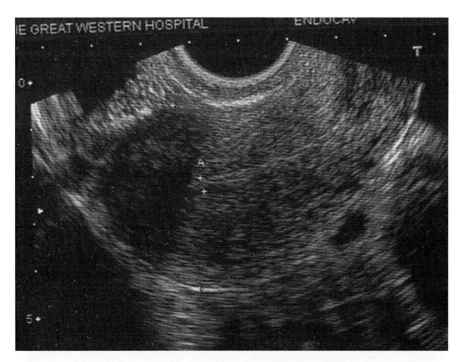

Figure 4.6 Postmenopausal endometrium seen on transvaginal ultrasound scan

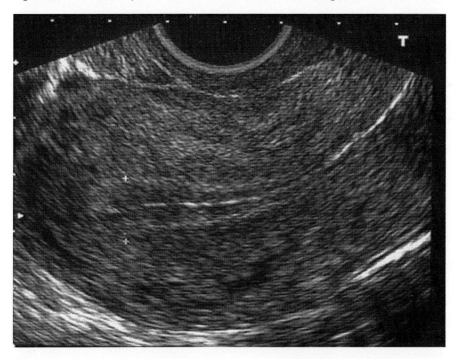

Figure 4.7 Preovulatory 'triple line' seen on transvaginal ultrasound scan

endometrial sampling methods are used a wide range of false-negative results occur.[17] The most consistent measurements are taken in the proliferative phase, when the endometrium is at its thinnest and most echolucent.[18] With all measurements of the endometrial echo, it is important to visualise it as a three-dimensional structure, to avoid missing focal irregularities. Three-dimensional ultrasound has an established role in the assessment of congenital uterine abnormalities[19] and in the future it may have a role in improving the visualisation of acquired conditions of the uterine cavity as well.

The endometrial outline should be regular and uninterrupted, whatever the thickness. A thick, secretory endometrium on unenhanced transvaginal ultrasonography will often disguise endometrial pathology. In contrast, a periovulatory 'triple line' endometrium (Figure 4.7) will offer the best unenhanced views of the uterine cavity. Most benign and cancerous lesions of the endometrium manifest themselves morphologically as polyps. These tend to be hyperechoic or cystic structures that distort the endometrial echo. Colour Doppler may demonstrate a single feeding blood vessel to the structure.

Uterine fibroids

Advances in the management of uterine fibroids have resulted in a need to provide accurate pretreatment information concerning their size, quantity and location. This information is especially important with the increasing use of minimally invasive techniques for fibroid resection. The appearances of myomas on ultrasound scanning are varied. Before the menopause, a myoma tends to be a well defined heterogeneous or hypoechoic uterine mass. TVUS can be an inaccurate method for mapping large uterine fibroids and magnetic resonance imaging (MRI) may provide added information. MRI is indicated when fibroid embolisation is planned because it allows the accurate assessment of fibroid shrinkage and the distinction of intramural fibroids from adenomyosis.[20] TVUS is used in conjunction with abdominal ultrasound scanning to ensure that pedunculated subserosal fibroids are not missed. Submucosal fibroids project into the uterine cavity and distort the endometrium. Their accurate classification allows selection for transcervical resection in appropriate cases. Fedele *et al.*[21] demonstrated the sensitivity of TVUS for the diagnosis of submucosal fibroids to be 100%, with a specificity of 94%. Hysteroscopy (outpatient) performed on the same population had a diagnostic sensitivity and specificity of 100% and 96%, respectively. The only criticism of TVUS in this study was its apparent inability to differentiate endometrial polyps from submucosal fibroids. Endometrial polyps tend to be hyperechoic structures, easily masked by a thick secretory endometrium. Performance of the scans during the proliferative phase makes the distinction between intracavity fibroids and polyps easier. A positive predictive value as high as 92% has been documented.[3]

Adenomyosis

This condition is characterised by the presence in the myometrium of endometrial glands and stroma, which may have a diffuse or focal distribution. It can be difficult to distinguish adenomyosis from intramural fibroids. This distinction is an important one to make because the definitive management of adenomyosis is hysterectomy, whereas fibroids can be treated with the conservation of the uterus. The reported sensitivity and specificity of TVUS in the diagnosis of diffuse adenomyosis is 80% and 74%, respectively, and 87% and 98% for focal lesions.[22] MRI scanning has, however, been shown to be significantly better than TVUS in the diagnosis of adenomyosis ($P < 0.02$).[9] For this reason, MRI remains the diagnostic modality of choice if fibroid embolisation is planned, but the use of MRI does add considerably to the overall cost of the treatment.

Saline sonohysterography

This technique involves the introduction of a sonographic negative contrast agent into the uterine cavity, to enhance routine transvaginal ultrasonography in the identification of uterine cavity pathology (Figure 4.8). The examination should ideally be performed in the proliferative phase of the menstrual cycle, once menstruation has ceased, in order to enhances the views of the uterine cavity.

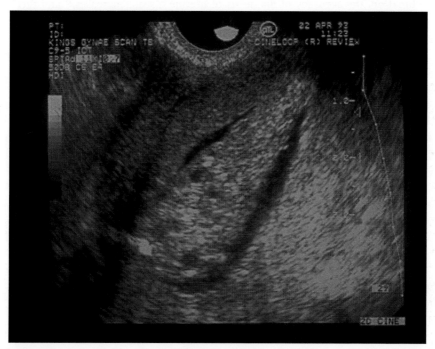

Figure 4.8 Saline hydrosongraphy demonstrating endometrial polypos (image reproduced with permission from Mr T Bourne)

Indications for saline hydrosonography are:

- Thickened endometrium
- Poor views of the endometrium owing to an axial position of uterus, and distortion of the uterine cavity by large fibroids
- Preoperative localisation, assessment of size and relation to the uterine cavity of submucous fibroids or endometrial polyps.

Overall failure rates range from 1.8%[23] to 4.6%.[24] There is no evidence to support the theoretical concern that instillation of fluid into the uterine cavity, either at hysteroscopy or saline sonohysterography promote dissemination of endometrial carcinoma.[25]

The primary diagnostic tool in the one-stop clinic

TVUS has been compared to hysteroscopy for the detection of intrauterine lesions.[26] In premenopausal women, the sensitivity and specificity of TVUS compared poorly with the results of outpatient hysteroscopy.[27] These findings have been supported by other studies.[28,29] There is, however, wide variation in the reported sensitivity and specificity of outpatient hysteroscopy, which can be as high as 94% and 89%, respectively.[30] When TVUS and hysteroscopy are used in combination, the accuracy of diagnosis of uterine disease increases,[31] and therefore TVUS is seen largely as an initial diagnostic method[32] that can be used prior to hysteroscopy.

The combination of TVUS with saline hydrosonography has, however, made ultrasound without hysteroscopy a potential first-line investigation.[3,6-8,33-36] One study[3] has shown that, compared with TVUS alone, TVUS plus saline hydrosonography increases the sensitivity from 67% to 87%, the specificity from 89% to 91%, the positive predictive value from 88% to 92% and the negative predictive value from 71% to 86%. These findings are supported by another study, which reported the sensitivity and the specificity of saline hydrosonography compared with those of hysteroscopy to be 90% and 83%, and 99% and 88%, respectively.[36] A randomised study comparing TVUS plus saline hydrosonography with office-based hysteroscopy for endometrial assessment has been carried out.[37] This study found a sensitivity and specificity of ultrasonography of 85% and 100%, respectively. The corresponding values for office-based hysteroscopy were 77% and 92%.

TVUS was acceptable to most women (95.7%[3]) attending the clinic. This finding is supported by data from a randomised trial,[37] which clearly demonstrated that more women preferred TVUS compared with hysteroscopy ($P < 0.001$). This is an extremely important observation when considering which investigation should be used as a first-line test. Furthermore, the availability of ultrasound at every consultation facilitates the incidental diagnosis of adnexal pathology, such as complex ovarian cysts. Incidental adnexal pathology was detected in 12 women (13.5%) attending an ultrasound-based one-stop clinic.[8]

Accreditation and training

A Special Skills module in 'Ultrasound Imaging in the Management of Gynaecological Conditions' is available from the RCOG and there are hysteroscopy training courses that are endorsed by the British Society for Gynaecological Endoscopy.

Conclusions

Abnormal uterine bleeding, whether it occurs in premenopausal or postmenopausal women, should be managed in a one-stop clinic that is set up to provide TVUS, hysteroscopy, and endometrial biopsy. A see-and-treat management philosophy can be offered to the majority of women. A critical appraisal of the scientific literature suggests that TVUS with endometrial sampling should be the primary diagnostic tool, and that hysteroscopy should be used selectively. By adopting these changes to the management of abnormal uterine bleeding, gynaecologists will shorten the care pathway for patients, and save resources for the hospital.

References

1. Vessey MP, Villard-Mackintosh L, McPherson K, Coulter A, Yeates D. The epidemiology of hysterectomy: findings in a large cohort study. *Br J Obstet Gynaecol* 1992;99:402–7.
2. Stabinsky SA, Einstein M, and Breen JL. Modern treatments of menorrhagia attributed to dysfunctional uterine bleeding. *Obstet Gynecol Surv* 1999;54:61–72.
3. Royal College of Obstetricians and Gynaecologists. *The initial management of menorrhagia. National evidence-based clinical guideline No. 1*. London: RCOG; 1998.
4. Royal College of Obstetricians and Gynaecologists. *The management of menorrhagia in secondary care. National evidence-based clinical guideline No. 5*. London: RCOG; 1999.
5. National Collaborating Centre for Women's and Children's Health. *Heavy Menstrual Bleeding*. Clinical Guideline. London: RCOG Press; 2007.
6. Scottish Intercollegiate Guidelines Network. *Investigation of post-menopausal bleeding. A national clinical guideline*. SIGN publication No. 61. Edinburgh: SIGN; 2002.
7. Gredmark T, Kvint S, Havel G, Mattsson LA. Histopathological findings in women with postmenopausal bleeding. *Br J Obstet Gynaecol* 1995;102:133–6.
8. Lidor A, Ismajovich B, Confino E, David MP. Histopathological findings in 226 women with post-menopausal uterine bleeding. *Acta Obstet Gynecol Scand* 1986;65:41–3.
9. Jones KD, Jermy K, Bourne TH. What is the correct primary diagnostic tool in the 'one-stop' clinic for the investigation of abnormal menstrual bleeding? *Gynaecological Endoscopy* 2002;11:27–32.
10. Holst J, Koskela O, von Schoultz B. Endometrial findings following curettage in 2018 women according to age and indications. *Ann Chir Gynaecol* 1983;72:274–7.
11. Stock RJ, Kanbour A. Prehysterectomy curettage. *Obstet Gynecol* 1975;45:537–41.

12. Koonings PP, Moyer DL, Grimes DA. A randomised clinical trial comparing Pipelle and Tis-u-trap for endometrial biopsy. *Obstet Gynecol* 1990;75:293–5.
13. Gimpelson RJ, Rappold HO. A comparative study between panoramic hysteroscopy with directed biopsies and dilatation and curettage. A review of 276 cases. *Am J Obstet Gynecol* 1988;158:489–92.
14. Smith P, Bakos O, Heimer G, Ulmsten U. Transvaginal ultrasound for identifying endometrial abnormality. *Acta Obstet Gynecol Scand* 1991;70:591–4.
15. Mendelson EB, Bohm-Velez M, Joseph N, Neiman HL. Endometrial abnormalities: evaluation with transvaginal ultrasonography. *AJR Am J Roentgenol* 1988;150:139–42.
16. Granberg S, Wikland M, Karlsson B, Norstrom A, Friberg LG. Endometrial thickness as measured by endovaginal ultrasonography for identifying endometrial abnormality. *Am J Obstet Gynecol* 1991;164:47–52.
17. Dijkhuizen FP, Brolmann HA, Potters AE, Bongers MY, Heintz AP. The accuracy of transvaginal ultrasonography in the diagnosis of endometrial abnormalities. *Obstet Gynecol* 1996;87:345–9.
18. Goldstein SR. Use of ultrasonohysterography for triage of perimenopausal patients with unexplained uterine bleeding. *Am J Obstet Gynecol* 1994;170:565–70.
19. Jurkovic D, Geipel A, Gruboeck K, Jauniaux E, Nutecci M, Campbell S. Three-dimensional ultrasound for the assessment of uterine anatomy and detection of congenital anomalies: a comparison with hysterosalpingography and two-dimensional sonography. *Ultrasound Obstet Gynaecol* 1995;5:233–7.
20. Goodwin SC, Walker WJ. Uterine artery embolisation for the treatment of uterine fibroids. *Curr Opin Obstet Gynecol* 1998;10:315–20.
21. Fedele L, Bianchi S, Dorta M, Brioschi D, Zanotti F, Vercellini P. Transvaginal ultrasonography versus hysteroscopy in the diagnosis of uterine submucous myomas. *Obstet Gynecol* 1991;77:745–8.
22. Fedele L, Bianchi S, Dorta M, Arcaini L, Zanotti F, Carinelli S. Transvaginal ultrasonography in the diagnosis of diffuse adenomyosis. *Fertil Steril* 1992;58:94–7.
23. Bernard JP, Lecuru F, Darles C, Robin F, de Bievre P, Taurelle R. Saline contrast sonohysterography as first-line investigation for women with uterine bleeding. *Ultrasound Obstet Gynecol* 1997;10:121–5.
24. Widrich T, Bradley LD, Mitchinson AR, Collins RL. Comparison of saline infusion sonography with office hysteroscopy for the evaluation of the endometrium. *Am J Obstet Gynecol* 1996;174:1327–34.
25. Devore GR, Schwartz PE, Morris JM. Hysterography: A 5-year follow-up in patients with endometrial carcinoma. *Obstet Gynecol* 1982;60:369–72.
26. Emanuel MH, Verdel MJ , Wamsteker K, Lammes FB. A prospective comparison of transvaginal ultrasound and diagnostic hysteroscopy in the evaluation of patients with abnormal uterine bleeding: clinical implications. *Am J Obstet Gynecol* 1995;172:547–52.
27. Pal L, Lapensee L, Toth TL, Isaacson KB. Comparison of office hysteroscopy, transvaginal ultrasonography and endometrial biopsy in evaluation of abnormal uterine bleeding. *JSLS* 1997;1:125–30. Erratum in: *JSLS* 1997;1:395.
28. Alcazar JL, Laparte C. Comparative study of transvaginal ultrasonography and hysteroscopy in postmenopausal bleeding. *Gynecol Obstet Invest* 1996;41:47–9.

29. Giusa-Chiferi MG, Goncalves WJ, Baracat EC, de Albuquerque Neto LC, Bortoletto CC, de Lima GR. Transvaginal ultrasound, uterine biopsy and hysteroscopy for postmenopausal bleeding. *Int J Gynaecol Obstet* 1996;55:39–44.

30. Indman PD. Abnormal uterine bleeding. Accuracy of vaginal probe ultrasound in predicting abnormal hysteroscopic findings. *J Reprod Med* 1995;40:545-8.

31. Feng L, Xia E, Duan H. Diagnosis of uterine disease by combined hysteroscopy and ultrasonography. *Zhonghua Fu Chan Ke Za Zhi* 1996;31:334-7.

32. Mortakis AE, Mavrelos K. Transvaginal ultrasonography and hysteroscopy in the diagnosis of endometrial abnormalities. *J Am Assoc Gynecol Laparosc* 1997;4:449-52.

33. Lev-Toaff AS, Toaff ME, Liu JB, Merton DA, Goldberg BB. Value of sonohysterography in the diagnosis and management of abnormal uterine bleeding. *Radiology* 1996;201:179-84.

34. Goldstein SR, Schwartz LB. Evaluation of abnormal vaginal bleeding in perimenopausal women with endovaginal ultrasound and saline infusion sonohysterography. *Ann NY Acad Sci* 1997;828:208-12.

35. Saidi MH, Sadler RK, Theis VD, Akright BD, Farhart SA, Villanueva GR. Comparison of sonography, sonohysterography, and hysteroscopy for evaluation of abnormal uterine bleeding. *J Ultrasound Med* 1997;16:587-91.

36. Bernard JP, Lecuru F, Darles C, Robin F, de Bievre P, Taurelle R. Saline contrast sonohysterography as first-line investigation for women with uterine bleeding. *Ultrasound Obstet Gynecol* 1997;10:121-5.

37. Timmerman D, Deprest J, Bourne T, Van den Berghe I, Collins WP, Vergote I. A randomized trial on the use of ultrasonography or office hysteroscopy for endometrial assessment in postmenopausal patients with breast cancer who were treated with tamoxifen. *Am J Obstet Gynecol* 1998;179:62-70.

5

Endometrial ablation

Kevin Jones

Introduction

In the previous chapter, we saw how the one-stop management philosophy can be applied to the investigation of women with menorrhagia. In this chapter, the conservative surgical treatment of this condition is described. The surgical treatment of women with menorrhagia who have no detectable pathology (i.e. women with dysfunctional uterine bleeding [DUB]) is called endometrial ablation. This is an office-based (outpatient) or daycase procedure, which destroys the lining of the uterus. The first-generation endometrial ablation techniques, such as trans-cervical electrosurgical resection or ablation, or the use of a neodymium:yttrium-aluminium-garnet laser, provided alternatives to hysterectomy and are carried out in the day surgery unit under spinal or general anaesthesia. These procedures are, however, being superseded by second-generation techniques, which require less technical skill to achieve uniform results and which are highly suitable for use in an outpatient gynaecology unit, in other words in the one-stop gynae-cology setting.[1]

Current methods of second-generation endometrial ablation

The use of second-generation devices generally involves destruction of the endometrium by heating or cooling. There are currently eight mechanisms and 12 instruments available. Only four of the devices, ThermaChoice® (Johnson & Johnson [corporation], New Brunswick, NJ, USA),[2] Vesta™ (Valleylab, Boulder, CO, USA),[3] MEA® (Microsulis, Denmead, UK)[4] and Hydro ThermAblator® (Boston Scientific Limited, Christ Church, Barbados, Figure 5.1a–b),[5] have been shown to be safe and effective in randomised clinical trials (RCTs) when compared with the first-generation techniques.

The Vesta™ system[3] is no longer available, and the remaining devices have been approved by the National Institute for Health and Clinical Excellence (NICE) in the UK. One other device, Cavaterm™ (Wallsten Medical SA, Morges, Switzerland) has been evaluated in an RCT of only 20 patients,[6] and it is currently undergoing evaluation in a larger RCT following initial evaluation studies by the same group.[7] Endometrial laser intrauterine thermal therapy (GyneLase®, Lumenis Ltd,

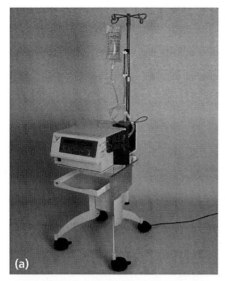 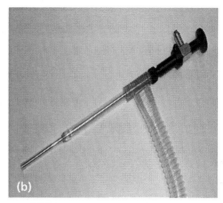

Figure 5.1 **(a)** The Hydro ThermAblator® and **(b)** integral hysteroscope

Yokneam, Israel),[8] Menostat™[9,10] (Rocket Medical, Watford, UK) and Her Option® office cryoablation therapy (American Medical Systems Gynecology Inc, Minnetonka, MN, USA)[11] are three instruments that have been evaluated in case series. In these evaluations, reported amenorrhoea rates ranged from 49% to 63% for the three different devices over variable follow-up periods. Case series have inherent limitations, which tend to make the success rates appear higher than in RCTs. The comparative amenorrhoea rates and mean reduction in menstrual scores from the RCTs are shown in Table 5.1.[2-5] The table also shows the performance of the Mirena® (Schering Health Care Ltd, Burgess Hill, UK) intrauterine contraceptive device (Figure 5.2) in a small RCT compared with transcervical electrosurgical resection.[12]

Table 5.1 Performance of second-generation endometrial ablation devices in randomised controlled trials

Device	Amenorrhoea rate (%)	Mean menstrual score (%)	Reference
ThermaChoice®	15	86	2
HTA®	40	77	5
Vesta™	32	94	3
MEA®	40	92	4
Mirena®	36	90	16

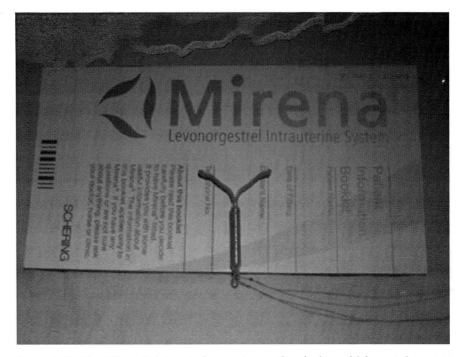

Figure 5.2   The Mirena® intrauterine contraceptive device, which contains levonorgestrel

The remaining instruments either have been evaluated in *ex vivo* studies, or the results are not reported in Medline-cited journals. In a modern health service it is incumbent upon us to practise evidence-based medicine. The devices evaluated in case series should therefore be subjected to RCTs prior to being introduced into routine clinical practice, and the devices rigorously evaluated in such trials should be the clinician's instrument of first choice. It is also becoming increasingly important to have NICE approval in order to introduce a new technology such as endometrial ablation into clinical service.

The four devices evaluated in RCTs

The ThermaChoice® System

The ThermaChoice® System uses hot fluid to destroy the endometrium. It consists of a catheter 16 cm in length and 4.5 mm in diameter with a latex balloon, housing a heating element, at its distal end. The balloon is inserted into the uterine cavity and filled with 5% dextrose in water. The treatment cycle is commenced when the fluid temperature reaches 87($\pm$5)°C and the cycle continues for 8 minutes. Treatment results in uniform coagulation of the endometrium by the transfer of heat through the balloon. ThermaChoice® was found to be equivalent to rollerball endometrial ablation in an RCT involving 245 women.[2] The procedure was performed in 47% of patients in an outpatient setting, without general anaesthesia, and there were no intraoperative complications noted amongst the women treated with the thermal balloon. Postoperatively, the balloon group reported one urinary tract infection and three cases of suspected endometritis; all resolved with oral antibiotics. At 12 months, the mean menstrual diary scores decreased by 86% (amenorrhoea rate 15%) and the dysmenorrhoea score decreased by 70%. With the rollerball technique, 92% of women reported a decrease in menstrual score, 27% reported amenorrhoea and the dysmenorrhoea score decreased by 75%. In this trial, 86% of the women were satisfied with the balloon treatment at 12 months. The only endometrial preparation used before treatment was a 3 minute curettage using a 5 mm suction curette.

The Vesta™ system

The Vesta™ system uses electrical energy to heat the endometrium and destroy it. It consists of an electrosurgical generator connected to a disposable handset. The handset, which is inserted into the uterine cavity, consists of an electrode carrier (air-filled balloon) with 12 flexible electrode plates covering its surface. The preset warm-up and treatment phases last 7 minutes and end automatically. In an RCT comparing Vesta™ with a combined transcervical loop resection and rollerball technique,[3] the mean menstrual diary scores at 12 months had decreased by 94% (amenorrhoea rate 32%) following the Vesta™ technique. In the electrosurgical group, the respective figures were 91%, and 40%. A total of 255 women were involved in the study. The Vesta™ procedure was carried out following a withdrawal bleed on the combined oral contraceptive pill. In this study, 83% of the women underwent the Vesta™ treatment in an outpatient setting, minor muscular fasciculation occurred during the Vesta™ treatment in 18 patients (12%), but in only one case was it necessary to halt the procedure. Patient satisfaction and changes in dysmenorrhoea scores were not recorded.

The MEA® system

The MEA® system uses microwave energy to destroy the endometrium. It consists of a computerised control unit and a set of applicators. The MEA® applicator is inserted into the uterine cavity, and supplies the microwave energy. The average treatment time for a uterus of normal size is less than 3 minutes. MEA® has been shown to be equivalent to transcervical resection in an RCT.[4] At 12 months, the mean menstrual diary and dysmenorrhoea scores decreased by 92% and 80%, respectively, with an amenorrhoea rate of 40%. In the electrosurgical group, the respective figures were 91% and 82%. Patient satisfaction and improvement in quality of life scores were high (70%) after 12 months. This study, which involved 240 women, was carried out in the UK, and all the procedures were done under general anaesthesia following endometrial preparation with a 5 week course of goseralin (Zoladex®, Astra Zeneca, Luton, UK). The main proponents of the device have considerable experience of using it under local anaesthesia in the outpatient setting, outside the context of an RCT.

The Hydro ThermAblator®

The Hydro ThermAblator® is an endometrial ablation device with an insulated sheath, which accepts a hysteroscope of up to a 3 mm in diameter. The device delivers heated saline solution at 90°C for 10 minutes into the uterus, at low pressure, to fully ablate the endometrium (Figure 5.1). The uterine cervix is dilated with a size 7 Hegar dilator and the insulated polycarbonate sheath (7.8 mm [24F]) and hysteroscope is then inserted into the uterine cavity. The polycarbonate sheath is positioned in the lower uterine segment so that the operator has a panoramic view of the uterine cavity. A tenaculum (e.g. Gimpelson) can be used to prevent leakage of fluid if there is an incomplete cervical seal. The Hydro ThermAblator® machine is then activated and room temperature saline solution is circulated under low pressure through the sheath and uterine cavity, enabling a diagnostic hysteroscopy to be performed prior to ablation of the endometrium. Gravity determines the maximum hydrostatic pressure and this pressure is achieved by setting the intravenous pole at a predetermined height. The maximum pressure reached is 50 mmHg, which is less than the opening pressure of the fallopian tubes (70–100 mmHg). There have been no incidences of reported tubal leakage and a maximum of 10 cm³ of fluid loss can occur before the flow of saline to the patient is stopped automatically and the operator is alerted. An aspiration pump evacuates the fluid and recirculates it through the device. The heater is then activated to allow gradual elevation of the temperature of the saline solution. Once the saline solution reaches a temperature of 90°C, the treatment cycle begins and continues for 10 minutes. At the end of the procedure, an automatic cool flush cycle is carried out using room temperature saline solution and the operator is prompted to remove the sheath at the completion of the treatment. The set-up and treatment cycles are microprocessor controlled, but the physician can interrupt treatment at any time if desired. The procedure was performed in 41% of patients in an outpatient setting, under local anaesthesia. The only intra-operative complications noted among the women treated with the Hydro ThermaAblator® were burns to the upper thigh and buttock in two women as a consequence of prolonged contact with the heated tubing that connected the control unit to the inflow channel of the hysteroscopic sheath. This problem has now been eliminated by a redesign of the insulation. At 12 months, the amenorrhoea rate was 40% and the mean decrease in menstrual bleeding score was 77%. These results persisted at 3 years following the procedure, when the amenorrhoea rate was 53% and the overall success rate was reported to be 94%, with a 98% patient satisfaction rate (Figure 5.3).[5]

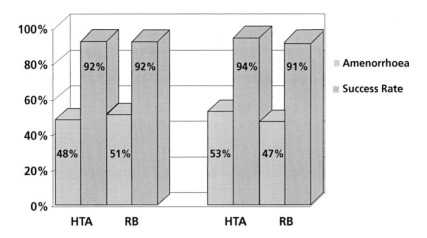

Figure 5.3   Outcome in patients treated with the Hydro ThermAblator® system (*n* = 177) compared with the rollerball technique (n = 85) at 12 months and 36 months after treatment.[5] HTA, Hydro ThermAblator®; RB, rollerball

Complications and postoperative care

In general, patients who have been treated with second-generation devices experience mild cramping pains, which are easily treated with simple analgesia, only in the immediate postoperative period. They may also have a watery, pink discharge, which should settle quickly. Postoperative endometritis is suggested by an offensive, blood-stained vaginal discharge and lower abdominal pain, and it can be treated with a course of antibiotics. With the exception of the Hydro ThermAblator®, all the second-generation devices are inserted into the uterine cavity blindly, rather than under hysteroscopic guidance, so if the uterus has been perforated the device could be activated in the pelvic cavity and could damage the adjacent organs. Although the UK Medicines and Healthcare products Regulatory Agency collects reports of complications associated with these second-generation devices, no national audit has been published. The clinical history of damage to the bowel, for example, would typically cause peritonism 24–48 hours after the patient has been discharged. Abdominal signs may be present and it is important that their significance is recognised. Hysterectomy may be necessary when there is failure to relieve the abnormal uterine bleeding, development of haematometra that cannot be relieved by cervical dilation alone, or severe endometritis. In the RCTs, the rate of hysterectomy ranged from 2% to 7% at 12 months. Menostat™ (a radiofrequency device) is, however, the only instrument that has been withdrawn by the UK Medicines and Healthcare products Regulatory Agency owing to the complications associated with its use.[10] Minimally invasive transcervical resection and ablation methods appear to leave islands of functional endometrium even if amenorrhoea results from the treatment, and concern exists about how they might behave if they underwent malignant change.[13] Guidelines to avoid this problem have been suggested.[14] For women who require hormone replacement therapy (HRT) to relieve climacteric symptoms, a no-bleed preparation seems the most appropriate.

Costs

With endometrial resection and ablation, direct and indirect costs are substantially less than those of hysterectomy, even taking into account treatment failures.[15] Units that already offer transcervical electrosurgical resection will have made a capital expenditure on the hysteroscopic equipment. There will, therefore, be little incentive for these departments to adopt new equipment, unless it allows the gynaecologist to treat women in an outpatient abnormal uterine bleeding clinic. For units that cannot offer endometrial ablation to women with DUB, however, these devices would be ideal. In the UK, the cost per treatment episode is broadly similar among all the second-generation devices. In order to establish such a service it is first necessary to write a business plan.

A model business plan for the introduction of the Hydro ThermAblator® device into a hospital (supplied by Boston Scientific, Natick, MA, USA) is shown in Appendix 5.2. This business plan (Appendix 5.1) presents a case for the establishment of an ambulatory gynaecology service, with a specific reference to endometrial ablation for DUB. It is a generic business plan so it can be applied to many areas of modern gynaecological practice that form part of the ambulatory gynaecology service.

Conclusions

On the basis of the highest standard of evidence, the Hydro ThermAblator®, Vesta™, MEA® and ThermaChoice® have been shown to be safe and effective treatments in appropriately selected women. The devices that are available commercially have NICE approval. It requires minimal training to use these devices, and they give equivalent results to the first-generation techniques. Family doctors and patients should be aware that these new technologies are now available to gynaecologists who have not been trained as advanced hysteroscopic surgeons, because they fill the therapeutic gap between drug therapy and hysterectomy for women with DUB and they can potentially be used in the one-stop gynaecology clinic.

References

1. Jones KD, McGurgan P, Sutton CJ. Second-generation endometrial ablation techniques. *Curr Opin Obstet Gynecol* 2000;12:273–6.

2. Meyer WR, Walsh BW, Grainger DA, Peacock LM, Loffer FD, Steege JF. Thermal balloon and rollerball ablation to treat menorrhagia: a multicenter comparison. *Obstet Gynecol* 1998;92:98–103.

3. Corson SL, Brill AI, Brooks PG, Cooper JM, Indman PD, Liu JH, *et al.* Interim results of the American Vesta™ trial of endometrial ablation. *J Am Assoc Gynecol Laparosc* 1999;6:45–9.

4. Cooper KG, Bain C, Parkin DE. Comparison of microwave endometrial ablation and transcervical resection of the endometrium for treatment of heavy menstrual loss: a randomised trial. *Lancet* 1999;354:1859–63.

5. Corson SL. A multicenter evaluation of endometrial ablation by Hydro ThermAblator and rollerball for treatment of menorrhagia. *J Am Assoc Gynecol Laparosc* 2001;8:359–67.

6. Romer T. Die therapie rezidivierender menorrhagien – Cavaterm-ballon koagulation versus roller-ball endometrium koagulation – eine prospektive randomiserte vergleichstudie. *Zentralbl Gynakol* 1998;120:511–4.

7. Hawe JA, Phillips AG, Chien PF, Erian J, Garry R. Cavaterm thermal balloon ablation for the treatment of menorrhagia. *Br J Obstet Gynaecol* 1999;106:1143–8. Erratum in: *BJOG* 2000;107:295.

8. Das Dores GB, Richart RM, Nicolau SM, Focchi GR, Cordeiro VC. Evaluation of Hydro ThermAblator® for endometrial destruction in patients with menorrhagia. *J Am Assoc Gynecol Laparosc* 1999;6:275–8.

9. Donnez J, Polet R, Squifflet J, Rabinovitz R, Levy U, Ak M, *et al.* Endometrial laser intrauterine thermo-therapy (ELITT): a revolutionary new approach to the elimination of menorrhagia. *Curr Opin Obstet Gynecol* 1999;11:363–70.

10. Phipps JH, Lewis BV, Roberts T, Prior MV, Hand JW, Elder M, *et al.* Treatment of functional menorrhagia by radiofrequency-induced thermal endometrial ablation. *Lancet* 1990;335:374–6.

11. Thijssen RF. Radiofrequency induced endometrial ablation: an update. *Br J Obstet Gynaecol* 1997;104:608–13.

12. Kittelsen N, Istre O. A randomized study comparing levonorgestrel intrauterine system (LNG IUS) and transcervical resection of the endometrium (TCRE) in the treatment of menorrhagia: preliminary results. *Gynaecological Endoscopy* 1998;7:61–5.

13. Rutherford TJ, Zreik TG, Troiano RN, Palter SF, Olive DL. Endometrial cryoablation, a minimally invasive procedure for abnormal uterine bleeding. *J Am Assoc Gynecol Laparosc* 1998;5:23–8.

14. Killick SR, Maguiess SD. Overview of menorrhagia. *Gynaecology Forum* 1997;2:2–5.

15. Valle RF, Baggish MS. Endometrial carcinoma after endometrial ablation: high-risk factors predicting its occurrence. *Am J Obstet Gynecol* 1998;179:569–72.

16. Hidlebaugh DA. Cost and quality-of-life issues associated with different surgical therapies for the treatment of abnormal uterine bleeding. *Obstet Gynecol Clin North Am* 2000;27:451–65.

Appendix 5.1

Model business plan for the introduction of the Hydro ThermAblator® device into a hospital (with permission from Boston Scientific, Natick, MA, USA)

This appendix gives only an example of a business plan. Its inclusion in this book does not represent the Royal College of Obstetricians and Gynaecologists' recommendation of the use of this business plan over any other.

Elsewhere Hospitals NHS Trust

Business Case for Adding HydroThermal Ablation to the Hospital's Treatment Portfolio for Menorrahgia™

Introduction

This business case sets out the key benefits of HydroThermal Ablation and the potential impact for the [local hospital] and for the people of [Somewhere].

At [date] Management Board meeting the Clinical Director for Women's Services tabled a case for funding the procedure in [Somewhere]. It was the Management Board's decision that the case should be presented to the [Somewhere] Primary Care Trust for consideration. However, it was the PCT's preference that this should be presented as part of the Service and Financial Framework (SaFF) process. It is therefore intended that the hospital management board should review the impact of this business case on overall capacity and local performance against access targets with a view to allocating waiting list money in [date.]

HTA: scientific and clinical background

In the UK, 5% of women of reproductive age will present to their family doctor annually seeking help for menorrhagia.[1] The majority of women have no underlying pathology detected after they have been investigated by the gynaecologist and they are then diagnosed as having dysfunctional uterine bleeding (DUB). The Royal College of Obstetricians and Gynaecologists (RCOG) reports that 42% of the 90 000 hysterectomies performed each year in the UK are for DUB.[2] To decrease the number of these operations, the RCOG has developed guidelines for the treatment of this condition.[3,4] All women should be offered medical therapy, the Mirena® intrauterine contraceptive device or an endometrial ablation procedure. Most recently the National Institute for Health and Clinical Excellence (NICE) has approved the use of the Hydro Thermal Ablator® (HTA) for treating women with DUB.[5] The HTA system has a number of advantages over the first generation techniques such as electrosurgical rollerball and other second generation ablation devices:

- Consistent results.
- Results are not dependent on skill or experience level of operator.
- Circulation of heated saline treats the entire uterine cavity.
- Visualisation of the cavity is possible throughout the procedure.
- Anatomical variations such as uterine cavity size, partial septate, partial bicornate uteri and fibroids can be treated.

The HTA is an endometrial ablation device with an insulated sheath, which accepts up to a 3-mm hysteroscope and delivers heated saline at 90°C for 10 minutes into the uterus at low pressure to fully ablate the endometrium. The technique is suitable for women with a diagnosis of DUB unresponsive to medical therapy, who have completed their families and wish to avoid a hysterectomy.

Treatment

The uterine cervix is dilated with a size-7 Hagar and the insulated polycarbonate sheath (7.8 mm/24 F) and hysteroscope is then inserted into the uterine cavity. The polycarbonated sheath is positioned in the lower uterine segment so that the operator has a panoramic view of the uterine cavity. A tenaculum (such as the Gimpelson) can be used to prevent leakage of fluid if there is an incomplete cervical seal. The HTA machine is then activated and room-temperature saline is circulated under low pressure through the sheath and uterine cavity, enabling a diagnostic hysteroscopy to be performed prior to ablating the endometrium. Gravity determines the maximum hydrostatic pressure and this is achieved by setting the IV pole at a predetermined height. This is equivalent to a maximum pressure of 50 mmHg, which is less than the opening pressure of the fallopian tubes (70–100 mmHg). There have been no incidences of reported tubal leakage and a maximum of 10 cc of fluid loss will stop the flow of saline to the patient connections and alert the operator. An aspiration pump evacuates the fluid and recirculates it through the device. The heater is then activated to allow gradual elevation of the saline temperature. Once the saline reaches a temperature of 90°C the treatment cycle begins and this lasts for 10 minutes. At the end of the procedure, an automatic cool flush cycle is carried out with room temperature saline and the operator is prompted to remove the sheath at the completion of the treatment. The set up and treatment cycles are microprocessor controlled, however the physician can interrupt treatment at any time if desired.

Anaesthesia and place of treatment

HTA cases have been performed under general or local anaesthesia, with and without conscious sedation. HTA cases have been performed in day surgery centres (ambulatory surgery centres) or on inpatient operating lists. They can also be performed in the outpatient clinic (offices procedures).

Results

The HTA device has been shown to be safe and effective in a randomised controlled trial comparing the HTA system with electrosurgical rollerball for the treatment of DUB.[6] There are a number of reasons for this:

- direct visualisation
- preoperative hysteroscopy to rule out intracavity pathology
- ensures correct placement of the device for effective treatment
- ensures correct placement of the device to avoid complications
- atraumatic introduction of the sheath under direct visualisation (less than 24 F)
- visualisation of uterine cavity before application of energy
- observation of uterine cavity during and after treatment
- controlled circulation of fluid
- confirmation of closed loop circulation with unheated fluid
- continuous monitoring of fluid volume and detection of 10 cc loss
- redundant heater control system to maintain temperature (in the trial, the beneficial effects at 12 months persist at 2 and 3 years; at 3 years following the procedure, the amenorrhoea rate was 53% and the overall success rate was reported to be 94% with a 98% patient satisfaction rate).[6]

Conclusion

The HTA system is a second-generation endometrial ablation device for the treatment of DUB. The amenorrhoea rate is 53% and the overall success rate 94%. It allows the operator to directly visualise the uterine cavity during the treatment, which promotes patient safety. The device has the potential to be used on large, irregular uterine cavities with submucous fibroids, polyps, and septae because it relies on freely circulating fluid.

Strategic context

The strategic vision set out in the NHS Plan provides the context for the development of services in Somewhere and is summarised in the following five components:

- providing a balanced range of services, which promote health & well being and tackle health inequalities.
- ensuring safe and high quality care with an increasing element of choice (the right care);
- which is fast and convenient (at the right time);
- as close to the home as possible (in the right place); and
- ending delays at all stages in the elective and emergency system.

This business case demonstrates how HTA will contribute to all five of the components of the Government's vision for the NHS.

The NHS Plan sets out the key targets that will need to be achieved in order to deliver the vision. In particular, HTA will contribute to the NHS Plan targets to reduce waiting times by increasing overall capacity for the hospital, reducing bed occupancy and by contributing to the infrastructure needed for services to be redesigned around the patients.

By [date], the Elsewhere Hospitals NHS Trust will be required to deliver the following key outcomes of the NHS Plan:

- booking all out-patients, day cases and in patients
- choice at the point of booking
- 6-month maximum wait inpatients
- 3-month maximum wait OP
- increased capacity
- increase in daycase rates to 75%.

The NHS Delivery Plan (2002) acknowledges that increased capacity will be needed to realise these benefits and recognises that bed occupancy rates should be reduced to an average 82%. The diagnostic and treatment centre programme is to be accelerated, demonstrating the importance of 'see and treat' service models, and more in-patients are to be treated as day cases to release hospital capacity.

PCTs have already begun to pay hospitals through an incentive system using a standard tariff based on national HRG benchmarks. Work will therefore need to be undertaken locally to drive unit costs closer to the UK average.

Hospitals are to be inspected by the Commission for Health Audit and Improvement CHAI and will continue to be allocated a star rating based on performance against an increasing range of Performance Assessment Framework (PAF) Indicators. CHAI will be given new powers to implement special measures if trusts do not perform at the expected level. The star rating of a trust currently affects its ability to access the NHS Performance Fund but in the future it will also affect the size of its baseline allocation. There are currently no PAF indicators directly relating to gynaecology. However, there are several new surgical technologies undergoing NICE appraisal and there has been recent media coverage that too many inappropriate hysterectomies are being carried out. It is likely that D&C and hysterectomy rates will be added to the indicators in the future. In addition, gynaecology activity affects the overall bed and theatre pool of the hospital and as a result has a direct impact on a range of key performance indicators including trolley waits and surgical access times.

The existing service

At [Quarter X; Year] local NHS Trust had [no. patients] cancelled as a result of a lack of beds. Medical outliers have frequently occurred on surgical wards and this has threatened to compromise the trust's ability to deliver waiting list reductions.

The hospital must make significant strides towards the [Year] targets. At [Quarter X; Year] the percentage of patients [% local data] who had waited more than 6 months for all inpatient procedures was higher than the local region and UK averages. Similarly, the percentage of patients [% local data] who had waited more than 6 months for a gynaecology procedure was significantly higher than local region and UK averages.

Waiting list	Somewhere NHS Trust	local region	UK average
All specialties			
Inpatient gynaecology			
Daycase gynaecology			

Percentage of patients waiting more than 6 months: [Complete with local data]

However, the table above shows that the percentage of patients [% local data] waiting more than 6 months for a daycase gynaecology procedure is lower in Somewhere than the local region and UK averages. This means that the contribution to reducing patients waiting over 6 months in gynaecology must primarily come from the inpatient lists. It will therefore be necessary to release more capacity in order to deliver more activity, or make better use of existing capacity.

At the end of [Quarter X, Y% of patients-local data] were waiting over 13 weeks for an outpatient appointment. The development of increased direct access and see and treat services would reduce this number.

Objectives

The objective of this business case is to fund the number of HTA per annum that would be required to convert 42% (1) of hysterectomies to a simple day case procedure, in order to:

- reduce the number of elective operations cancelled by the hospital
- increase day case rates
- free up capacity in main theatres and wards for waiting list initiatives
- reduce the overall unit cost of treatment
- shorten the whole treatment process for patients
- speed up recovery and return to work for patients
- deliver the principles of governance and controls assurance.

Benefits and success criteria

1. Saving in 'bed days'
The gynaecology department carried out [X hysterectomies-local data] for DUB, between [dates]. It is suggested that 42% (1) of these patients could have been

treated by HTA and approximately 4% (6) of these patients would have gone on to require a hysterectomy. An abdominal procedure has an average bed stay of 6 days [local data]. The net saving in 'bed days' of converting 42% [of X hysterectomies-local data], with a 4% (6) failure rate to HTA, with a zero bed stay, over a year would be:

Worked example:

For every 100 hysterectomies performed, 42 could be converted to an HTA procedure. Of these, 40.3 are successful and 1.7 (4% failure rate) go onto require a hysterectomy.

Therefore: 40.3 (no. HTAs) x 6 (length of hospital stay)

= 242 bed days saved/year/100 hysterectomies.

2. Operating lists saved

HTA procedures take an average of 35 minutes [local data] (time in theatre, i.e. speculum to speculum time) and hysterectomies take around 90 minutes [local data] (time in theatre). Therefore, five HTA procedures can be undertaken in a 3-hour session compared with two hysterectomies. The net annual saving in converting the hysterectomies to HTA procedures would be:

Worked example:

For every 100 hysterectomies performed, 42 could be converted to an HTA procedure. Of these, 40.3 are successful and 1.7 (4% failure rate) go on to require a hysterectomy.

Therefore: 40.3 hysterectomies requires 20 operating lists (rate: two per 3 hours)

40.3 HTAs requires eight operating lists (rate: five per 3 hours)
= 12 operating lists saved/year/100 hysterectomies

- The inpatient theatre capacity released could be used to reduce the in patient waiting list in gynaecology and/or overall by the equivalent of Y major procedures per annum [local data] (depends on time in theatre / procedure). Beds released could be used for waiting list initiatives or to accommodate rising emergency admissions and to reduce the risk of hospital cancellations of elective patients.
- Since HTA can be carried out in a day case or outpatient environment, it is a procedure that lends itself to booked admissions.
- For the patients who would not require a follow up hysterectomy, the impact of the change would be a significantly shorter wait for treatment, a day case or out-patient attendance rather than a 6-day hospital stay, and a 1–2 day return to normal functioning compared with 2–8 weeks.

- HTAn has NICE approval,[5] is a low-risk procedure and is highly consistent with the requirements of clinical governance and controls assurance.
- The clinical, hospital and patient benefits of HTA are highly consistent with the requirements of the NHS Plan and the new NHS Delivery Plan. The change will further the trust's position against key access targets and will bring the trust further in line with regional and national averages for patients waiting over 6 months.
- HTA can be conducted by a nurse practitioner and therefore supports the development of new and innovative roles in the NHS.

Cost

The list price for HTA disposable procedure kits is £395. The capital equipment will be provided on a loan basis subject to procedure numbers. The key differences between the hysterectomy and HTA procedures are calculated top down as follows:

Operating differences	Abdominal hysterectomy (A)	HTA (B)	Cost difference per case (B–A)
Disposable procedure kits	Nil	375	375
Theatre time*	252	101	151
Bed days	1164	0	1164
TOTAL	1416	476	Saved 940

* Average cost of a theatre session @ NHS Trust is £504, so the cost assumes two hysterectomies or five HTAs per list. The average cost of a surgical bed day is £194 **[local data]**.

In real terms, the estimated annual cash-releasing effect of transferring 42% (1) of patients to HTA, with a 4% (6) failure rate is calculated to be:

Worked example:

40.3 (no. HTA's) x £940 (cost difference per case)

= £37,882 saved/year/100 hysterectomies.

In reality, it is unlikely that the hospital will wish to take up the option to release cash. A preferred option might be to spend £ZZZ K per annum [local data] and generate the capacity to treat more major cases [local calculation of no.] on a waiting list initiatives.

If HTA were to be provided in outpatients, this would free up capacity to treat even more in patient and day cases [local calculation of no.].

Implementation

It is proposed that for the first year the service would be provided in the daycase environment and later transferred to the outpatient environment. The gynaecology team are establishing a dedicated hysteroscopy service, using cancer modernisation money, and the same facility could be used for HTA. In some centres in the UK, 'see and treat' centres have been established, incorporating direct access hysteroscopy followed by same day HydroThermal Ablation treatment for selected patients.

References

1. Vessey MP, VillardMackintosh L, McPherson K, Coulter A, Yeates D. The epidemiology of hysterectomy: findings in a large cohort study. *Br J Obstet Gynaecol* 1992;99:402–7.
2. Seth A, Stabinsky ME, and Breen JL. Modern treatment of menorrhagia attributed to dysfunctional uterine bleeding. *Obstet Gynaecol Surv* 1998;54(1):61–72.
3. Royal College of Obstetricians and Gynaecologists. The Initial Management of Menorrhagia.Evidence-Based Clinical Guideline No. 1. London: RCOG Press; 1998.
4. Royal College of Obstetricians and Gynaecologists. *The Management of Menorrhagia in Secondary Care.* Evidence-Based Clinical Guideline No. 5. London: RCOG Press; 1999.
5. Nationasl Institute for Health and Clinical Excellence. Interventional Procedural Guidance 51. March 2004; ref No 496.
6. Corson SL. A multicentre evaluation of endometrial ablation by Hydro ThermalAblator and rollerball for treatment of menorrhagia. *J Am Assoc Gynecol Laparosc* 2001;8(3):359–67.

Acknowledgements

Supported by an unconditional educational grant from Boston Scientific.

6

Urogynaecology: urinary incontinence and genital prolapse

Natalia Price and Simon Jackson

Introduction

The assessment and investigation of the gynaecological patient are rapidly moving away from the operating theatre and ward environment and into the outpatient department. This move has been fuelled by the demands of the patient and the clinician for a rapid, accurate diagnosis, with the minimum of investigations and invasive procedures, as well as by the economic constraints of inpatient admission.

Urinary incontinence and genital prolapse are common and debilitating conditions. Estimates of their prevalence vary considerably according to the different populations studied and the various definitions used. Whichever estimates are used, however, urinary incontinence and genital prolapse are undoubtedly common in apparently healthy women. Urinary incontinence may be defined as 'the complaint of any involuntary leakage of urine'.[1] Not everyone with incontinence is sufficiently bothered by the symptoms to want help. Furthermore, there is reluctance to seek help and only about one-third of regularly incontinent women discuss their problem with a nurse or general practitioner.

In this chapter, we first describe what investigations and management can be undertaken at the primary care level for women with symptoms of urinary incontinence and genital prolapse, and we suggest referral guidelines that are vital for the effective use of secondary care resources. We then describe what can reasonably be covered in a single visit to a specialist urogynaecology clinic, the so-called the 'one-stop urogynaecology clinic'.

Primary care management

A general practitioner sees women with a range of symptoms including urinary frequency, daytime urgency and nocturia, incomplete bladder emptying, poor urinary stream, recurrent cystitis and bladder pain. Many of these symptoms coexist, but the majority of women will complain of urinary incontinence. All women with lower urinary tract symptoms must have a basic assessment, which

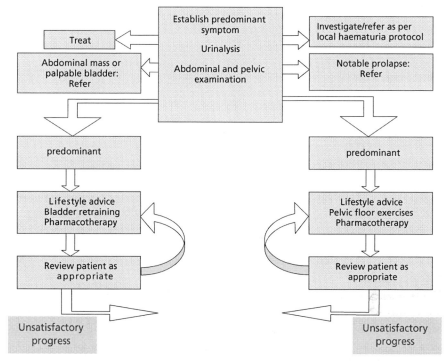

Figure 6.1 Female urinary incontinence: primary care management guidelines

should include a clinical history and examination, urinalysis and a self-completed urinary diary. Such an assessment can be performed within the primary care setting. Many women do not need to progress any further and can be managed with simple advice and treatment. Conservative measures that may be undertaken include decrease of caffeine consumption, reduction or increase of fluid intake, pelvic floor exercise, bladder drill, treatment of urinary tract infection and the prescription of anticholinergic drugs. Guidelines for primary care management are illustrated in the flow chart in Figure 6.1.

Initial assessment

History
It is important to prioritise any problems by identifying the predominant symptom. Such symptoms may include urinary incontinence, increased daytime frequency, nocturia, urgency, dysuria, bladder pain, haematuria, incomplete emptying, poor urinary stream and hesitancy. In addition to these symptoms, the clinician should enquire about colorectal symptoms and genitourinary prolapse.

When obtaining the woman's history, the aim should be to explore possible aetiological factors and to enquire about neurological disease, past obstetric trauma and previous gynaecological and urological surgery. A good evaluation of the clinical history will include enquiries about the impact of the disease on quality of life by asking how the symptoms affect aspects of daily life and social, personal and sexual relationships.

Questionnaires have been developed to allow lower urinary tract symptoms, their severity and quality of life to be measured in a reproducible way, without bias from the interviewer.[2,3] These questionnaires can be used in primary care settings, enabling standardisation of symptoms assessment, prioritisation of symptoms and measurement of the severity and impact of disease.

Clinical examination

Clinical examination should include an abdominal examination and a bimanual examination. Neurological assessment of the lower limbs and perineum is required if a neurological cause is suspected. Vaginal examination should include an assessment of descent of the urethra and bladder neck on straining, mobility of the anterior vaginal wall and concurrent uterovaginal prolapse.

Urinary diary

The frequency of micturition and leakage episodes can be assessed using a daily diary. This is a simple and practical method of obtaining information on voiding behaviour. A frequency/volume chart records the time and volume of all voids over specific period, which should include day and night and be of at least 24 hours' duration. The median value for voiding in asymptomatic women is seven to eight times in 24 hours and the frequency of micturition tends to increase with age.

Urinalysis and urine culture

Urinary tract infection can mimic any lower urinary tract condition, causing frequency, urgency and incontinence. Urine microscopy and culture is the diagnostic gold standard but reagent strip testing of urine for leucocyte esterase and nitrates is sensitive and provides a cheaper screening method. Bacteriological analysis is reserved for those with a positive screening test result.

Haematuria diagnosed by dipstick should always be confirmed by microscopy on a midstream sample of urine before further evaluation is undertaken. Urine should also be sent for cytological analysis. Urine cytology can detect transitional cell carcinoma, with sensitivity varying from 20% to 90% depending on the tumour grade.

Many urology departments now have one-stop haematuria clinics that aim to achieve diagnosis at a single outpatient visit (Box 6.1). Available investigations include urine cytology, renal tract ultrasonography, intravenous urography and flexible cystourethroscopy. Women with significant proteinuria, red cell casts or renal insufficiency should be referred to a nephrologist.

Box 6.1 Summary for haematuria

- All women with haematuria merit investigation with urine microscopy, culture, cytology and biochemistry; renal tract ultrasound and plain abdominal X-ray should also be performed.
- Frank or microscopic haematuria in those aged over 40 years or in younger, high-risk women should be investigated as above and a cystoscopy should be performed.
- Further investigations with intravenous urography and/or computed tomography imaging may be required.

Management

Management of predominant stress urinary incontinence

Conservative therapy can be initiated in primary care. The symptoms of stress incontinence can be treated through, for example, adjustment of lifestyle, pelvic floor exercise or pharmacotherapy.

Encouraging the cessation of smoking, treating chronic cough conditions, providing advice on weight reduction and rectifying exacerbating conditions such as constipation can often help to reduce the severity of symptoms.

The aim of pelvic floor exercise is to promote the woman's awareness of her pelvic floor muscles and to improve their contractility and coordination. Whenever possible, an appropriately trained physiotherapist should make an assessment of the pelvic floor musculature.

Pelvic floor exercise is an appropriate first-line treatment for most women. A proportion will not benefit, however, and in these women additional investigation and treatment should not be delayed. Pelvic floor exercise has been compared with no treatment for incontinent women in two randomised controlled trials.[4] Women performing pelvic floor exercise were more likely to be dry or mildly incontinent (61%) than those receiving no treatment (3%). Exercise needs to be continued on a long-term basis to prevent the recurrence of symptoms.

Several classes of drug could be beneficial in the treatment of stress urinary incontinence. Estrogens have been proposed as a treatment for stress incontinence; many women feel their incontinence gets worse or commences around the time of the menopause. Trials do not, however, support their use, [5-7] although there is some evidence that estrogens used in conjunction with α-agonists may be beneficial.

At present, attention is focusing on a potent selective norepinephrine and serotonin reuptake inhibitor (duloxetine). Preliminary clinical studies have confirmed its efficacy in the treatment of stress incontinence.[8] A one-month therapeutic trial of duloxetine in a selected group of patients with symptoms suggestive of stress urinary incontinence can be initiated at the primary care level. If no improvement in symptoms is observed after 1 month, however, treatment should be stopped and referral to specialist clinic should be considered.

Box 6.2 Pharmacological agents used in the treatment of urinary incontinence

Antimuscarinics

- Oxybutynin hydrochloride
- Tolterodine tartrate
- Propiverine hydrochloride, solifenacin succinate and trospium chloride

Tricyclic antidepressants

Estrogens.

Management of predominant urgency and urge urinary incontinence

Urgency, with or without urge incontinence, and usually with frequency and nocturia, can be described as 'overactive bladder syndrome'.[1] This diagnosis can be strongly suspected from the woman's history and frequency/volume chart. The primary treatment is behaviour modification and pharmacotherapy with anticholinergic drugs. Before empirical treatment, the woman should complete a urinary diary and have urine tested for blood and infection, in order to exclude factors such as malignancy, untreated diabetes and polydipsia. Urgency, frequency and urge urinary incontinence can be treated using behaviour modification techniques, bladder training and pharmacotherapy.

Reduction of fluid intake, if the urinary diary suggests it is excessive, and cutting caffeinated products out of the diet will often have a dramatic effect. Simple behavioural advice such as this may be all that is required to cure frequency and urgency. The three main components of bladder training are patient education, timed voiding with systematic delay in voiding, and positive reinforcement. The woman should be asked to resist the sensation of urgency and void according to a timetable. A self-completed urinary diary should be used to monitor the times of voids. Continence rates of up to 90% have been reported but the corresponding cure rates could be considerably lower than this.[9]

Pharmacological suppression (Box 6.2) of detrusor overactivity with anticholinergic agents (antimuscarinics) is the most widely used treatment for this condition.[10] Antimuscarinic drugs are the mainstay for pharmacological treatment of detrusor overactivity. Their tolerance is limited, however, by adverse effects, which include dry mouth, blurred vision, dizziness, constipation, nausea and insomnia. As these drugs are essentially safe, it would seem reasonable clinical practice to commence a short course of empirical treatment in cases where detrusor overactivity is suspected clinically. If symptoms are not improved after 1 or 2 months of anticholinergics, the woman should be referred to a specialist clinic.

Secondary care: the one-stop urogynaecology clinic

If the initial management of lower urinary tract symptoms during primary care has failed or, in cases where specific indications (e.g. substantial prolapse, hae-

---

Box 6.3 Summary of the indications for urodynamic assessment

- Complex, mixed urinary symptoms (urge incontinence, stress incontinence, frequency)
- Symptoms of stress urinary incontinence
- Symptoms suggestive of detrusor overactivity, unresponsive to pharmacotherapy
- Voiding dysfunction with incomplete bladder emptying
- Neuropathic bladder disorder (videourodynamics preferred).

---

maturia, abdominal or pelvic mass, urinary retention etc.) are present, then more extensive investigations would be required and the woman should be reviewed in a one-stop urogynaecology clinic. This visit would include consultation with a specialist urogynaecologist, including review of the history and clinical examination, and urodynamic investigation. If the primary care guidelines outlined above are followed, almost everyone referred for secondary care will require urodynamic assessment.

The concept of a one-stop urogynaecology clinic implies that the findings of these investigations will be reviewed during the consultation, and that the appropriate treatment or management plan can be initiated on the same day.

Urodynamic assessment

Urodynamic investigations include uroflowmetry, post-void residual measurement and cystometry, all of which can be performed easily in an outpatient clinic. The indications for urodynamic assessment are set out in Box 6.3.

Uroflowmetry and ultrasonography

The symptoms of dysfunctional voiding are non-specific but, if abnormal voiding is suspected, it is important to carry out further investigation of flow, using uroflowmetry, and of post-void residual urine, by ultrasonography. These tests are particularly important when investigating recurrent urinary tract infections or before commencing treatment of women with anticholinergic preparations. Furthermore, uroflowmetry is also an essential preliminary test before proceeding with formal cystometry.

Cystometry

Cystometry aims to explain a clinical problem in pathophysiological terms. It involves measurement of the pressure versus volume relationship of the bladder during filling and voiding and it is a useful test of bladder function. This investigation is simple, accurate and easy to perform, taking between 15 and 20 minutes, which is feasible in an outpatient setting.

Booking for surgical treatment

In cases where conservative treatment has been tried during primary care and has failed, and when urodynamic investigation has subsequently confirmed the presence of stress incontinence, a woman can be booked to receive the appropriate surgical procedures during a first outpatient consultation. The Royal College of Obstetricians and Gynaecologists' Guideline No.35[11] recommends that, 'since the best chance of surgical "cure" for stress incontinence is successful primary surgery, surgical treatment should only be considered after a period of conservative treatment from a specialist therapist has been offered and rejected, or has failed'. The choice of surgical procedure should be made according to the underlying pathophysiology of the stress incontinence.

Secondary care: daycase surgery

Stress urinary incontinence

The surgical procedures outlined below can be performed as daycase surgery and are therefore potentially suitable for one-stop therapy.

Periurethral bulking injections

Currently, the two most commonly used injectable preparations for bulking are collagen (Contigen®, Bard, Crawley, W Sussex) and silicone rubber (Macroplastique®, Uroplasty Inc, Minneapolis, MN, USA). Injections are usually given with cystoscopic guidance, although urethral guides have been developed to allow blind insertion of Macroplastique® in an outpatient setting (Figure 6.2). Injection can be performed under local anaesthetic. The technique is minimally invasive and has extremely low complication rates. Reported cure rates vary but may be as low as 7% for objective cure. According to Jarvis's meta-analysis in 1994,[12] the success rate of periurethral bladder-neck injection in the treatment of primary urodynamic stress incontinence is 45.5%, and 57.8% for recurrent stress incontinence. Efficacy is often short-lasting, particularly if an absorbable product such as collagen is used, and reinjection is frequently required. Although the injectable materials are expensive and the results mediocre, the procedure has a low complication rate and a quick recovery phase. These advantages make the technique particularly suitable for frail, elderly people.

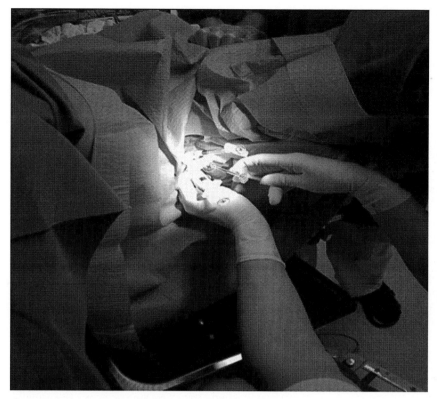

Figure 6.2 Insertion of bulking agent using a urethral guide

Tension-free vaginal tape

The advent of tension-free vaginal tape (TVT) has changed the practice of many clinicians and insertion of a TVT sling is rapidly becoming the primary operation for genuine stress incontinence. This operation is performed using a minimally invasive technique that was originally described as an 'ambulatory procedure carried out under local anaesthesic'.[13]

Various transvaginal retropubic slings are available from different manufacturers. The sling is inserted transvaginally, aiming to provide support at mid-urethral level (Figure 6.3). A trocar is passed retropubically, bilaterally, and cystoscopy should be performed after the insertion of each trocar to detect perforation of the bladder. Once the tape is positioned, tension is applied while the woman coughs.

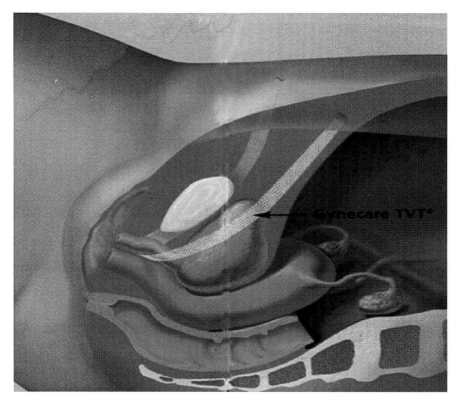

Figure 6.3   The tension-free vaginal tape is inserted to support the mid-urethra

Although the use of TVT is relatively new, increasing numbers of cohort studies are being reported. The subjective and objective results of a 6-month randomised trial that compared TVT with Burch colposuspension showed similar continence rates for both procedures.[14] Complete dryness in each group was 36% and 28%, respectively. Large cohort analysis has shown a continence rate of 80% and an improvement rate of 94%.[15] In the UK, the use of TVT has now received approval from the National Institute for Health and Clinical Excellence.[16]

Transobturator tape insertion

Transobturator tape (TOT) (Figure 6.4) is similar to TVT but a different technique is used to insert the tape. It can be inserted under spinal, general or local anaesthesia. The tape is positioned without tension under the junction between the mid and distal urethra. The main difference between this procedure and TVT insertion is that the retropubic space is not entered and cystoscopy is not routinely required.

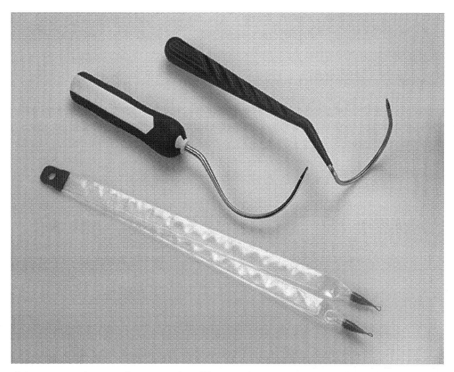

Figure 6.4 Obtryx® (Boston Scientific, Maple Grove, MN, USA) transobturator tape

The National Institute for Health and Clinical Excellence Interventional Procedures Advisory Committee has given a provisional recommendation for TOT, stating that the current evidence on the safety and efficacy of transobturator tape insertion for stress urinary incontinence appears adequate to support the use of this procedure, provided that the normal arrangements are in place for consent, audit and clinical governance. The lack of long-term data was emphasised, particularly when comparing this procedure with TVT insertion.[17]

Surgical treatment for overactive bladder

Surgery is recommended for intractable detrusor overactivity only when medical and behavioural therapy has failed. The mainstay of surgical management is augmentation cystoplasty, although cystodistension and bladder denervation have been used.

New developments such as neuromodulation and botulinum toxin injection may offer hope for the future. Botulinum toxin, injected cystoscopically into detrusor muscle in five to 30 different locations, while sparing the trigonum, works by paralysis of the muscle. There is preliminary evidence, based on uncontrolled, observational studies, that botulinum A toxin injection into detrusor muscle inhibits the symptoms of bladder overactivity.[18-20] Efficacy is short-lived and injections probably require repetition every 3–6 months. Additional studies to determine ideal doses, dosing intervals, safety and effectiveness are warranted. When more clinical data become available, botulinum toxin injection could potentially be performed on a daycase basis.

Genital prolapse

Daycase surgery for genital prolapse under local anaesthetic has recently been tried and advocated. The advantages are clear: a shorter hospital stay and an early return home. Monga and colleagues[21] studied women with at least a grade 2 cystocele, rectocele or both, and repaired these under local anaesthetic with fascial techniques; 67–88% of the women were cured at a median follow-up of 30 months.

In our practice, we perform daycase anterior colporrhaphy for moderate anterior vaginal wall prolapse, but not posterior colporrhaphy, owing to the more complex nature of the latter procedure. We have observed that there is relatively little postoperative pain, allowing early mobilisation and discharge from hospital.

Conclusion

In this chapter, we have described what investigations and management can be undertaken at the primary care level for women with symptoms of urinary incontinence and genital prolapse. We have also suggested appropriate referral guidelines for general practitioners. We have then considered what can reasonably be covered in a single visit to a specialist one-stop urogynaecology clinic. Although it would clearly not be possible to solve all the problems of all the patients during a single visit to a urogynaecology clinic, for very many women it would undoubt edly result in a shorter care pathway. Provided that the referral guidelines are followed properly by general practitioners, it should also result in the more efficient use of secondary care resources. We therefore recommend the one-stop urogynaecology clinic for audited trial.

References

1. Abrams P, Cardozo L, Fall M, Griffiths D, Ulmsten U, van Kerrebroeck P, *et al.* The standardisation of terminology of lower urinary tract function: report from the Standardisation Sub-committee of the International Continence Society. *Neurourol Urodyn* 2002;21:167–78.
2. Jackson S, Donovan J, Brookes S, Eckford S, Swithinbank L, Abrams P. The Bristol Female Lower Urinary Tract Symptoms questionnaire: development and psychometric testing. *Br J Urol* 1996;77:805–12.
3. Avery K, Donovan J, Peters TJ, Shaw C, Gotoh M, Abrams P. ICIQ: a brief and robust measure for evaluating the symptoms and impact of urinary incontinence. *Neurourol Urodyn* 2004;23:322–30.
4. Berghmans LC, Hendriks HJ, Bo K, Hay-Smith EJ, de Bie RA, van Waalwijk van Doorn ES. Conservative treatment of stress urinary incontinence in women: a systematic review of randomized clinical trials. *Br J Urol* 1998;82:181–91.

5. Jackson S, Shepherd A, Brookes S, Abrams P. The effect of oestrogen supplementation on post-menopausal urinary stress incontinence: a double-blind placebo-controlled trial. *Br J Obstet Gynaecol* 1999;106:711–8.

6. Fantl JA, Cardozo L, McClish DK. Estrogen therapy in the management of urinary incontinence in postmenopausal women: a meta analysis. First report of the Hormones and Urogenital Therapy Committee. *Obstet Gynecol* 1994;83:12–8.

7. Moehrer B, Hextall A, Jackson S. Oestrogen for urinary incontinence in women. *Cochrane Database Syst Rev* 2003;(2):CD001405.

8. Cardozo L, Drutz HP, Baygani SK, Bump RC. Duloxetine response and onset of action in women with severe stress urinary incontinence awaiting continence surgery. Int J Gynaecol Obstet 2003;83:34.

9. Wallace SA, Roe B, Williams K, Palmer M. Bladder training for urinary incontinence in adults. *Cochrane Database Syst Rev* 2004;(1):CD001308.

10. Nabi G, Cody JD, Ellis G, Herbison P, Hay-Smith J. Anticholinergic drugs versus placebo for overactive bladder syndrome in adults. *Cochrane Database Syst Rev* 2006;(4):CD003781.

11. Royal College of Obstetricians and Gynaecologists. Surgical treatment of urodynamic stress incontinence. Clinical Guideline No. 35. London: RCOG; 2003.

12. Jarvis GJ. Surgery for genuine stress incontinence. *Br J Obstet Gynaecol* 1994;101:371–4.

13. Ulmsten U, Henriksson L, Johnson P, Varhos G. An ambulatory surgical procedure under local anesthesia for treatment of female urinary incontinence. *Int Urogynecol J Pelvic Floor Dysfunct* 1996;7:81–6.

14. Ward KL, Hilton P. A randomised trial of colposuspension and tension-free vaginal tape for primary genuine stress incontinence. *BMJ* 2002;325:67–75.

15. Ulmsten U, Falconer C, Johnson P, Jomaa M, Lannér L, Nilsson CG, *et al.* A multicenter study of tension-free vaginal tape (TVT) for surgical treatment of stress urinary incontinence. *Int Urogynecol J Pelvic Floor Dysfunct* 1998;9:210–3.

16. National Institute for Health and Clinical Excellence. Urinary incontinence: the management of urinary incontinence in women. Clinical guideline CG040. London: NICE; 2006.

17. National Institute for Health and Clinical Excellence. International procedures overview of transobturator foramen procedures for stress urinary incontinence. London: NICE; 2005.

18. Reitz A, Stohrer M, Kramer G, Del Popolo G, Chartier-Kastler E, Pannek J, *et al.* European experience of 200 cases treated with botulinum-A toxin injections into the detrusor muscle for urinary incontinence due to neurogenic detrusor overactivity. *Eur Urol* 2004;45:510–5.

19. Flynn MK, Webster GD, Amundsen CL. The effect of botulinum-A toxin on patients with severe urge urinary incontinence. *J Urol* 2004;172:2316–20.

20. Rapp DE, Lucioni A, Katz EE, O'Connor RC, Gerber GS, Bales GT. Use of botulinum-A toxin for the treatment of refractory overactive bladder symptoms: an initial experience. *Urology* 2004;63:1071–5.

21. Kuhn A, Gelman W, O'Sullivan S, Monga A. The feasibility, efficacy and functional outcome of local anaesthetic repair of anterior and posterior vaginal wall prolapse. *Eur J Obstet Gynecol Reprod Biol* 2006;124:88–92.

7

Infertility

Valentine Akande, Elinor Medd and Kevin Jones

Introduction

Infertility is defined by World Health Organization as the diminished or absent ability to conceive or produce an offspring. Most couples plan on having a baby and for the majority this happens within a reasonable length of time. For one in six couples this does not occur, however, and help may be needed to assess their condition and initiate treatment.

Within the past two decades, owing to notable advances, the majority of infertile couples can be offered some form of treatment that improves their chance of conceiving. A decision on what form of treatment is most suitable, however, requires a diagnosis, which involves various investigations and examinations. On reaching a diagnosis appropriate counselling, prognosis and treatment can be offered. Ideally a diagnosis should be reached in as short a time as possible.

Management of the newly referred infertile couple is often frustrating for the patient, general practitioner and clinician alike for the following reasons:

- There is often a delay in the waiting time from referral to consultation, regardless of the cause of infertility
- At the first consultation, a working diagnosis or prognosis is difficult to establish because the results of all essential preliminary investigations are often not available.

Almost all gynaecologists see and investigate infertile women or couples, but the Royal College of Obstetricians and Gynaecologists has recommended that optimal care is best provided in a dedicated environment – a fertility clinic. The introduction of a one-stop fertility clinic would help solve some of these problems. Its aim would be to cut down the waiting time from referral to diagnosis and initiation of treatment, or the waiting time for referral to an assisted conception unit.

A one-stop management service would reduce costs because there would be fewer clinic appointments, and unnecessary invasive and expensive procedures would potentially be avoided. Furthermore, a cost-effective system for the investigation of the infertile couple would allow funding to be directed towards treatments for couples.

Although the concept of one-stop clinics is not new to the specialty, its application to 'fertility patients' has been limited to focusing on an individual aspect such as endoscopy[1] or imaging assessment of the female pelvis.[2] In this chapter, we present a streamlined care pathway suitable for most infertility referrals.

Guidelines for investigation

Differences of opinion exist in relation to what investigations are the most appropriate. With the recent publication of guidelines, by the UK's National Institute for Health and Clinical Excellence (NICE),[3] for the assessment and treatment for people with fertility problems, a consensus now exists. This fertility guideline is a compilation of evidence-based recommendations. The principles of care state there should be couple-centred management, access to evidence-based information and involvement of a specialist team.

Organisation of the service

The infrastructure required to set up the one-stop service includes a dedicated clinic area, with reception seating and, preferably, with relevant information points. Dedicated staff should be familiar with the equipment being used and the management approach set out in the NICE guidelines. Receptionists arrange appointments, collate results and update patient information efficiently. Nursing staff should chaperone couples during the consultation and act as their advocate if appropriate. The lead clinicians should be subspecialists with an interest in reproductive medicine or infertility. It would therefore be expected that the team would have an up-to-date, evidence-based approach to clinical management.

Given that the timing of fertility tests is often related to the menstrual cycle, a phlebotomy service that includes an out of hours service should be available. The clinic would require facilities for ultrasonography, hysterosalpingo contrast sonography (HyCoSy) or transvaginal hydrolaparoscopy (THL; Fertiloscopy®, Soprane, Lyon, France). It is also important to have access to local virology, haematology and biochemistry laboratories and methods of transportation of specimens on the same day. Equipment within the consultation room itself should be of a standard arrangement, ensuring adequate light source by the examination couch. It must be possible to darken the room during ultrasonography procedures.

Referral

In order to pursue a one-stop management philosophy for couples seeking fertility treatment, it is important to establish the criteria for referral to secondary care. NICE guidelines state that referral for investigation of infertility in secondary centres should occur following 2 years of regular unprotected sexual intercourse with no conception. Referral to a one-stop clinic would not be appropriate for couples with a pre-existing (confirmed) diagnosis for their infertility, for example severe endometriosis that requires specialist laparoscopic surgery.

Couples should be offered initial lifestyle advice, which may assist conception prior to referral. Such lifestyle modifications include having unprotected sexual intercourse every 2–3 days, drinking less than 1–2 units of alcohol per week (women) or less than 3–4 units of alcohol per week (men), discontinuation of smoking, aiming to achieve a body mass index of 19–29, and avoidance of occupational hazards. Folic acid supplementation and cervical screening should also be recommended as part of preconceptual preparation.

Method and protocols

Following referral, an appointment to be seen in the clinic is sent to couples. Prior to this appointment, couples are sent a pack of written information, containing details of the process of events, an explanation of the investigations and an overview of fertility problems and management. Included in the patient information pack are forms for blood tests and semen analysis, with specific instructions. The three main areas of assessment are sperm, ovulation and tubal defects. The basic investigations are listed in Table 7.1. These tests should be requested in all patients prior to their formal consultation in the one-stop fertility clinic.

Table 7.1 Pre-clinic investigations				
Gender	**Test**	**Timing**	**Area of assessment**	**Comments**
Female	Serum FSH/LH	Day 2–5	Ovulation or ovarian reserve	All women
Female	Serum chlamydia antibody titre	Any time	Tubal damage	All women
Female	Serum testosterone/SHBG	Any time	Ovulation or PCOS	All women
Female	Serum prolactin	Any time	Ovulation	If periods irregular
Female	Serum TSH	Any time	Ovulation	If periods irregular
Female	Serum progesterone	Luteal phase	Ovulation	All women
Female	Cervical swab/serum chlamydia antibody titre	Any time	Infection	All women
Male	Seminal fluid analysis	Any time	Sperm	All men

FSH, follicle stimulating hormone; LH, luteinising hormone; PCOS, polycystic ovary syndrome; SHBG, sex hormone binding globulin; TSH, thyroid stimulating hormone

Rubella, hepatitis and HIV screening should also be offered to all women as part of preconceptual 'good practice' that is in the interests of the offspring. The couple should be asked to complete a detailed, structured self-history questionnaire before attendance at the clinic. This saves the time normally taken to obtain a history during the consultation. It also provides essential information that allows appropriate further investigations or treatment to be instigated. It may also avoid inappropriate referral.

A request is made for series of standard investigations, some of which need to be done at specific times of the menstrual cycle (Table 7.1). The information obtained in the results of these tests is essential for an effective consultation. In women with periods that occur infrequently, drug treatment (progesterone, 5 mg three times daily for 5 days) may need to be started in primary care to initiate a withdrawal bleed in order to time the investigations.

At the one-stop consultation the couple's medical notes, including the self-completed history sheet and test results, are collated and reviewed by the clinician. If preliminary investigations reveal a problem such as azoospermia, then further assessment in the one-stop clinic would be inappropriate. The couple should be directed to an assisted conception unit or to an andrology clinic. A physical examination and a transvaginal ultrasound scan (TVUS) are performed to assess the pelvic anatomy.

The gold standard for the assessment of tubal factors in infertility is laparoscopy. This technique is performed under general anaesthesia in the day-surgery theatre; however, transvaginal hydrolaparoscopy under sedation in the office environment is now possible. The microlaparoscope is introduced into the pelvis through the pouch of Douglas. It is helpful to undertake a screening test in those women most likely to have tubal damage. This is done by serum chlamydia antibody testing, which can also help select the patients most likely to have severe tubal damage for assessment of their pelvis by formal laparoscopy or THL. In women with positive serology and high antibody titre, laparoscopy is the most appropriate method of tubal assessment.[4] This procedure should preferably be carried out by a gynaecologist trained in advanced laparoscopic surgery so that a see-and-treat procedure is possible.

In women who are at low risk of tubal damage and pelvic adhesions, investigations to assess tubal patency include HyCoSy, THL and hysterosalpingography. The choice of investigation depends on the availability of expertise and equipment within the unit. From a pragmatic point of view and within the remit of most one-stop clinics, HyCoSy would be the investigation of choice.

Initial discussion of diagnosis and management of the couple is undertaken at this stage, in light of all the available results. A plan of management is then instigated and treatment initiated or agreed upon. Supplementary investigations are arranged and, if necessary, referral to an assisted conception unit.

Practical techniques

The investigations performed in the one-stop clinic should involve evaluation of the female genital tract and, in particular, the patency of fallopian tubes. Sperm and ovulatory function would have already been established by prior laboratory analysis.

For tubal assessment, NICE recommends hysterosalpingography or HyCoSy. Laparoscopy and dye hydrotubation is advised if there is a suspected co-morbidity such as endometriosis or previous pelvic infection. Clearly, hysterosalpingography (Figure 7.1) needs to be carried out in a radiology department, and laparoscopy with dye hydrotubation (Figure 7.2) in the day-surgery unit under general anaesthesia. These techniques cannot, therefore, be performed in the one-stop outpatient setting. Fertiloscopy® (THL), on the other hand, in some European centres is becoming an established procedure that allows assessment of the fallopian tubes and parts of the pelvis[5] (Figure 7.3).

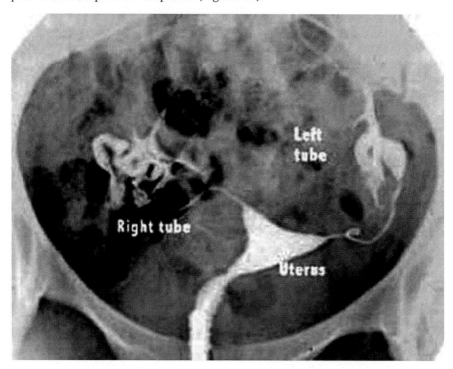

Figure 7.1 A hysterosalpingogram demonstrating the pelvic organs

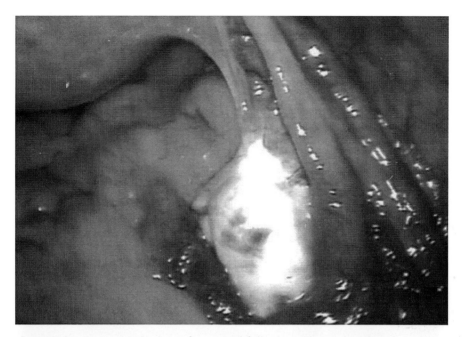

Figure 7.2 Laparoscopic view of a normal fallopian tube and ovary

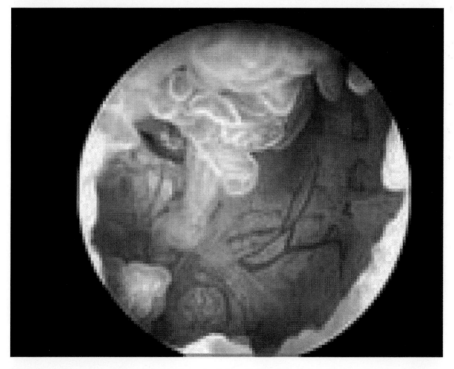

Figure 7.3 View of the fimbrial end of the fallopian tube during Fertiloscopy®
(transvaginal hydrolaparoscopy)

Pelvic ultrasound

Pelvic ultrasound can be used to assess the uterine cavity and the morphology of the ovary. The transvaginal approach provides the clearest imaging of the female genital tract. The uterus is assessed for fibroids, endometrial regularity and size. Assessment of the ovaries can enable the diagnosis of polycystic ovaries, normal (follicular) ovarian cysts (Figure 7.4) and hyperstimulated ovaries with multiple ovarian cysts or endometriomas (Figure 7.5). The antral follicle count or ovarian volume may be used as an indicator of ovarian reserve. The presence of congenital abnormalities, such as a bicornuate uterus, can be seen on ultrasound (Figure 7.6) and in some cases pelvic adhesions can also be suspected from the ultrasound appearance (Figure 7.7).

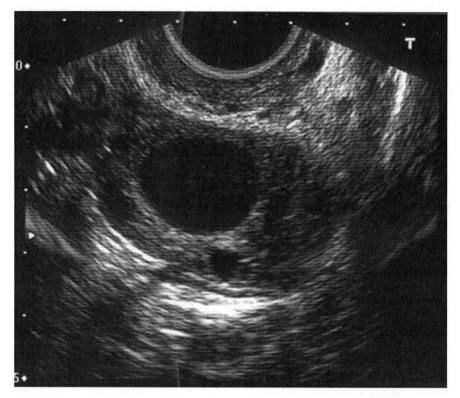

Figure 7.4 A normal ovary with a follicular cyst seen on transvaginal ultrasound scan

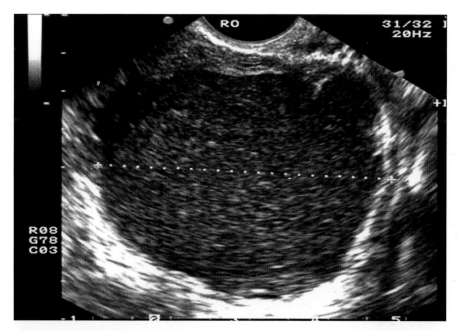

Figure 7.5 Endometrioma seen on transvaginal ultrasound scan (Photograph reproduced with permission from Mr Tom Bourne)

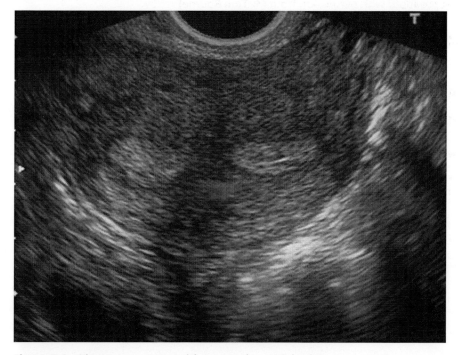

Figure 7.6 Bicornuate uterus with two endometrial echoes seen on 2-dimensional transvaginal ultrasound scan

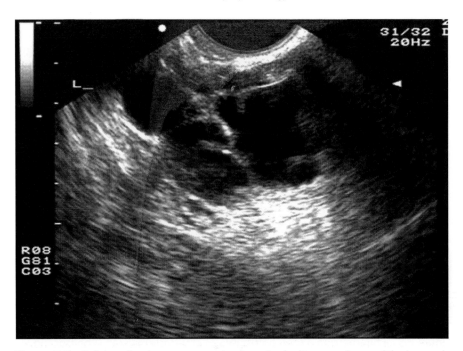

Figure 7.7 Pelvic adhesions seen on transvaginal ultrasound scan (Photograph reproduced with permission from Mr Tom Bourne)

Table 7.2 Comparisons between Fertiloscopy® and HyCoSy

Technique	Limitations	Benefits
Fertiloscopy®	Time consuming (mean 33 min[8]) Operator dependent Visceral injury and infection risk 0.25%[5] Sterile technique needed Ambulatory setting	Suitable for one-stop clinic Only local anaesthetic is required Well tolerated compared with hysterosalpingography Views of pelvic peritoneum and tubes possible Can diagnose adhesions and endometriosis Biopsies can be taken to diagnose endometriosis
HyCoSy	Difficult to visualise length of fallopian tube Not possible to diagnose endometriosis or adhesions Operator dependent	Suitable for one-stop clinic Well tolerated compared with hysterosalpingography Sensitive screen for tubal patency Immediate result No anaesthetic required

Assessment of tubal patency

Central to a one-stop management strategy is the ascertainment of tubal patency or occlusion. The two most commonly used techniques that can be used in a one-stop setting are HyCoSy or THL (Figure 7.3). The choice of technique used is dependent on operator experience and competence and the availability of equipment at the centre. A higher operative risk is associated with THL compared with HyCoSy, although the potential to take biopsies and perform treatment are potential benefits of THL. The limitations and benefits of each of these techniques are listed in Table 7.2. Prior to procedures for the assessment of tubal patency, antibiotics are given if an active infection has been detected by the cervical swabs undertaken during the preliminary investigations.

Hysterosalpingo contrast sonography

This technique combines a basic TVUS and a test of tubal patency using contrast media. The procedure can be performed without local anaesthetic in the outpatient setting. The contrast medium (Echovist®, Schering, Berlin, Germany; Figure 7.8) is prepared immediately before use. A catheter is then introduced through the cervix and the contrast medium is injected into the uterine cavity while a TVUS is performed. The procedure is well tolerated compared with hysterosalpingography.[6] A limitation of HyCoSy is that it is rarely possible to visualise the complete

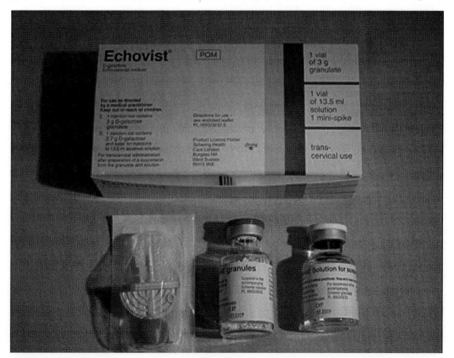

Figure 7.8 The contrast medium (Echovist®) used for HyCoSy studies

---

Box 7.1 The stages of Fertiloscopy®

- Hydropelviscopy is the key step of Fertiloscopy®. It consists of the introduction of 200 cm³ saline into the pelvis via the vagina and then insertion of a telescope (up to 4 mm diameter) into the pelvis via the vagina through an FTO 1.40™ balloon introducer (Soprane, Lyon, France; Figure 7.3). The pelvic organs can then be examined with high precision in this aqueous environment.
- A dye test can be carried out by the injection of methylene blue into the uterus using a specific FH 1.29™ balloon introducer (Soprane, Lyon, France). This test allows tubal patency to be tested.
- Salpingoscopy involves insertion of the telescope into the fimbria, followed by the ampulla, of each fallopian tube in order to explore the tubal mucosa.

---

length of the fallopian tube in a single scanning plane.[7] There is the potential for three-dimensional imaging to be used to overcome this problem and permit analysis of the flow of contrast through the tube.

Fertiloscopy® (transvaginal hydrolaparoscopy)

Fertiloscopy® permits visual exploration of tubo-ovarian structures under local anaesthetic and sedation (Figure 7.3 and Box 7.1). It is therefore highly suitable for use as part of the one-stop management philosophy. The woman is placed in a lithotomy position (Trendelenburg tilt is not required), the vagina is cleaned with antiseptic solution, local anaesthetic injected and the cervix grasped and manipulated in order to expose the posterior vaginal fornix. A small-diameter telescope (4 mm) is introduced through the posterior vaginal fornix. The peritoneal cavity is distended with saline, permitting visualisation of adhesions and endometriosis, and allowing demonstration of tubal patency with methylene blue dye. The procedure takes approximately 10–15 minutes to complete. Another advantage of THL is that it can be combined with outpatient hysteroscopy, fimbroscopy and salpingoscopy. The combination of THL with hysteroscopy has been shown to be a reliable technique, which provides more information and is better tolerated than hysterosalpingography.[8]

The contraindications to Fertiloscopy® are obstructive disorders of the pouch of Douglas, especially fixed retroversion, bulky posterior fibroids or large-volume ovarian cysts; infiltration of the recto-vaginal septum; or obliteration of the pouch of Douglas by endometriosis.

Complications that may occur are rectal injury (the injury is subrectal and does not require any special treatment other than increased patient surveillance for 48 hours and antibiotic cover), infection and false passage. The limitation of Fertiloscopy® is that the anterior part of the uterus and the vesico-uterine cul-de-sac cannot be visualised.

Interpretation of fertility investigations

The results of all investigations should be discussed, giving the couple reassurance that the whole process is thorough and complete. When an abnormality is discovered, it is vital that the prognosis of natural conception is discussed along with possible treatment options. A provisional plan should be drawn up as to future care. Some couples may need time, however, to evaluate their options and consider the appropriate plan for themselves. Under these circumstances a further consultation may be required.

Training for the one-stop fertility service

The main areas of specialist training required for medical staff working in a one-stop clinic for the investigation of the infertile couple are TVUS, THL and outpatient hysteroscopy. Specialist accreditation can be achieved via the British Society for Gynaecological Endoscopy, who run accredited training in laparoscopy and hysteroscopy. Training in Fertiloscopy® is available in several centres in Europe (e.g. the Centre de Recherche et d'Etude de la Stérilité, Lyon, France) and the USA.

Conclusions

The one-stop clinic approach to the investigation of the infertile couple enables a structured assessment of fertility during a single outpatient visit. Assessment of the fallopian tubes and uterine cavity can be undertaken and the results of prior investigations taken into account to provide the couple with a treatment plan and prognosis. Couples with infertility will benefit from a shorter interval between initial referral and diagnosis because the one-stop clinic will facilitate rapid referral to an assisted conception unit, if necessary. Referral to the clinic is appropriate only if there is no previously known diagnosis that accounts for the infertility.

References

1. Brosens I, Gordts S, Valkenburg M, Puttemans P, Campo R, Gordts S. Investigation of the infertile couple: when is the appropriate time to explore female infertility? *Hum Reprod* 2004;19:1689–92.
2. Strandell A, Bourne T, Bergh C, Granberg S, Thorburn J, Hamberger L. A simplified ultrasound based infertility investigation protocol and its implications for patient management. *J Assist Reprod Genet* 2000;17:87–92.
3. National Institute for Health and Clinical Excellence. Fertility: assessment and treatment for people with fertility problems. Clinical guideline CG011. London: NICE; 2004.
4. Akande VA, Hunt LP, Cahill DJ, Caul EO, Ford WC, Jenkins JM. Tubal damage in infertile women: prediction using chlamydia serology. *Hum Reprod* 2003;18:1841–7.

5. Gordts S, Campo R, Puttemans P, Verhoeven, H Gianaroli L, Brosens J, *et al.* Investigation of the infertile couple: a one-stop outpatient endoscopy-based approach. *Hum Reprod* 2002;17:1684-7.

6. Watrelot A, Dreyfus JM, Andine JP. Evaluation of the performance of fertiloscopy in 160 consecutive infertile patients with no obvious pathology. *Hum Reprod* 1999;14:707-11.

7. Cicinelli E, Matteo M, Causio F, Schonauer LM, Pinto V, Galantino P. Tolerability of the mini-pan-endoscopic approach (transvaginal hydrolaparoscopy and minihysteroscopy) versus hysterosalpingography in an outpatient infertility investigation. *Fertil Steril* 2001;76:1048-51.

8. Kelly SM, Sladkevicius P, Campbell S, Nargund G. Investigation of the infertile couple: a one-stop ultrasound-based approach. *Hum Reprod* 2001;16:2481-4.

8

Early pregnancy units and emergency gynaecological services

Chris Pearce and Kevin Jones

Introduction

The early 1990s saw the inception of the first early pregnancy units (EPUs),[1] which were established to treat women with complications of pregnancy in the first trimester. It was recognised that EPUs were an efficient way of organising the services compared with traditional care pathways. Demand on the service has increased in recent years with the use of home pregnancy kits and the consequent confirmation of pregnancies at extremely early gestations. In recent years, many units have developed into comprehensive early pregnancy care facilities, incorporating day care for women undergoing surgical or medical interventions. Prompt diagnosis and treatment in a dedicated EPU facility ensures that the woman receives continuity of care, which is frequently led and delivered by nursing staff. Anxiety is minimised and ongoing health is ensured through support and monitoring.

More recently, this concept has been expanded to incorporate all emergency gynaecological care that previously presented to an accident and emergency unit. Women with acute gynaecology problems should ideally be seen in emergency gynaecology units (EGUs), which are set up and run along similar lines as the EPU.

National targets

The National Service Framework for Children, Young People and Maternity Services[2] is clear in its aim of providing patient-centred care with the identification and appropriate management of relevant social, medical and psychiatric problems. This framework follows a one-stop assessment, diagnosis and management ethos as set out in the NHS Plan.[3] The National Strategy for Sexual Health and HIV[4] is comprehensive in its mission to improve health, sexual health and wellbeing, with a particular focus on the achievement of fewer undiagnosed infections and lower rates of unintended pregnancies. This challenge must be taken up by EPUs and EGUs, where it must be recognised that although the bulk of the activity may occur in primary care, secondary care has an important part to play in health education and promotion, contraception, prevention of high-risk sexual behaviours, and the detection and prevention of sexually transmitted infections.

Organisation of the service

Setting

Although the setting for EPUs and EGUs varies between hospitals, the requirements remain the same. There is much debate whether such units should be based within gynaecology or obstetrics but the most important factors are the skills and attitudes of the staff involved. Certainly, women have voiced their concerns at being within an environment that promotes normal pregnancy, with overt baby noise and pictures, when they are experiencing early pregnancy problems with an unknown outcome.

The location of the EPUs and EGUs is fundamental because units located close to or within the gynaecology ward allow continuity of out of hours service, which is provided by the ward team. Essential infrastructure consists of a reception area with dedicated staff who have access to information technology such as patient databases, a clinical examination room with the facilities to undertake minor procedures, an ultrasound room equipped with a machine that is less than 5 years old,[5] a designated waiting area with toilet facility, and spaces for beds or trolleys to accommodate women who need to recline. The aim is to create an environment not only for the administration of care to women with gynaecological problems but also to promote sexual health and wellbeing. In short, a first class service for women.[6]

Access

The gold standard would be a unit that is open every day, with the specialist staff available to provide appropriate care. Resource restrictions do not, however, allow this level of service. A unit will typically be staffed between 08.00 hours and 20.00 hours from Monday to Friday, and on Saturday morning. During these times nurses with advanced practice training should be available. In some units an appointment system is in place. Out of hours, if the EPU or EGU is located correctly, the unit can be covered by the senior nursing staff who are on duty on the gynaecological ward. There should always be available an identified member of the medical team and a lead clinician at consultant level. The unit requires a dedicated ultrasound service with facilities for the requisite laboratory investigations. Same-day biochemical estimation of beta human chorionic gonadotrophin (ßhCG) level is an integral part of the one-stop culture. Through cross-boundary work with primary care and the production of guidelines for referral, emergency gynaecology referrals can also be seen in the unit. This achievement stems from reinforcement of the philosophy that most emergency gynaecology referrals do not need to be seen immediately unless they require acute intervention. A reduction in the number of out of hours attendees has thus been seen.

There should be a 24 hour telephone helpline number, which is supported by the unit in opening hours or by the gynaecology ward out of hours. Women feel more able to manage their condition at home if they are able to call for specialised advice at any time, should they run into difficulty. The helpline is therefore a key factor in the arrangement of services.

Method of referral

All women who are attending for the first time must be referred from another healthcare professional. There is inevitably a degree of self-referral, particularly by women who have had problems in a previous pregnancy.

Staffing of the unit

The unit should be run as a multidisciplinary service. There should be a lead consultant as well as a nursing lead who supervises the work of nurse practitioners and middle grade medical staff. In different units various individuals perform the transvaginal ultrasound scan (TVUS). This service could be provided by dedicated sonographers or trained nurses and doctors. Clerical staff are vital for any busy unit, to enter data onto information systems, obtain notes and fax results immediately to general practitioners, freeing nursing and medical staff to provide clinical care.

Education and training

Even if the EPU or EGU is led by nursing staff, it is essential that junior doctors participate in care in order to gain the necessary skills in a supervised capacity. The nurses within the unit should have advanced skills and experience in gynaecological nursing plus counselling skills that enable them to take a brief history, obtain and order tests, make a diagnosis and treat problems in early pregnancy. Only qualified individuals should undertake TVUS (Box 8.1).

Box 8.1 Staff required for the provision of ultrasound scanning in the early pregnancy unit or emergency gynaecology unit

- Radiographers, midwives or nurses with the Postgraduate Diploma in Medical Ultrasound
- Radiologists with ultrasound training and experience as recommended by the Royal College of Radiologists
- Obstetricians, gynaecologists or radiologists who have completed the joint ultrasound training scheme of the Royal College of Obstetricians and Gynaecologists and the Royal College of Radiologists.

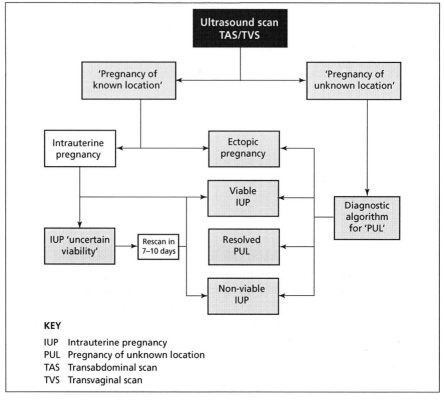

Figure 8.1 Diagnostic algorithm for early pregnancy loss

Clinical indications

Referral guidelines for primary care and other healthcare professionals should be available and distributed regularly with updated information. These guidelines should be multidisciplinary and should be based on the Royal College of Obstetricians and Gynaecologists guidelines and current evidence of best practice.

Management protocols

Early pregnancy loss

Management strategies for early pregnancy loss are based on clinical and investigative findings (Box 8.2) and the strategies should be discussed with the woman. The majority of early pregnancy complications can be managed in the ambulatory care environment, achieving high levels of patient satisfaction (Figure 8.1).

TVUS is used to confirm fetal viability and to measure growth (Figures 8.2 and 8.3). It is also used to make the diagnosis of a miscarriage or an ectopic pregnancy.

Box 8.2 Findings and management strategies for early pregnancy loss

- History
- Clinical findings
- Ultrasound findings
- Biochemical investigation
- Treatment and management plan
- Health education and promotion.

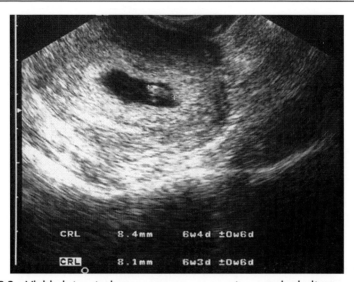

Figure 8.2 Viable intrauterine pregnancy seen on transvaginal ultrasound scan at 6 weeks' amenorrhoea

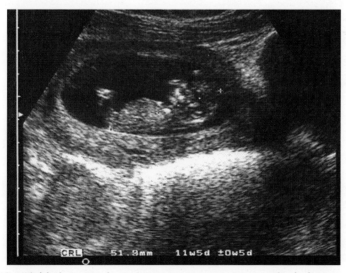

Figure 8.3 Viable intrauterine pregnancy seen on transvaginal ultrasound scan at 11 weeks' amenorrhoea

If the gestation sac on TVUS is more than 20 mm in diameter with no yolk sac, this finding is classified as an anembryonic pregnancy or early embryonic demise (Figure 8.4). If the crown-to-rump length is at least 6 mm and there is no fetal cardiac activity, or if the crown-to-rump length is more than 6 mm with no change at the time of a repeat scan 7 days later, this is classified as a missed miscarriage or early fetal demise (Figure 8.5).

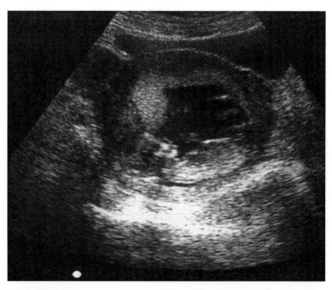

Figure 8.4 Anembryonic pregnancy (early embryonic demise) seen on transvaginal ultrasound scan

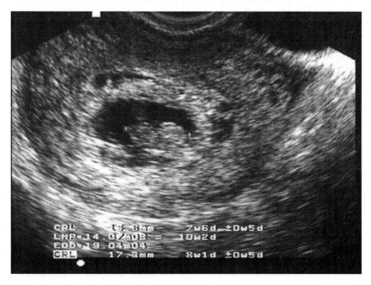

Figure 8.5 Missed miscarriage (early fetal demise) at 10 weeks' amenorrhoea seen on transvaginal ultrasound scan

Many women prefer expectant management and the literature suggests that up to 80% of women can be managed in this way with no subsequent impairment in cumulative conception rates or pregnancy outcome.[7,8] An alternative is medical evacuation, which is performed using oral mifepristone followed 48 hours later by oral or vaginal misoprostol. Evidence suggests that vaginal misoprostol may be more effective.[9,10] Surgery may be the best choice for those women who feel unable to cope with not knowing when the miscarriage may take place or for those who are bleeding heavily and are in pain. All women should be asked for consent for the taking of a chlamydial detection swab, as set out in the Royal College of Obstetricians and Gynaecologists guideline for the management of early pregnancy loss.[11]

Products of conception

It is usual practice to submit products of conception for histological examination to exclude ectopic pregnancy and gestational trophoblastic disease. It is essential, however, that all products of conception are disposed of sensitively. All products typically undergo a cremation organised by the pastoral department of the hospital trust. This practice enables a meaningful conversation when parents question the whereabouts of the products of conception evacuated in theatre or passed during their stay on the unit.

Ectopic pregnancy

Highly sensitive pregnancy tests and the ease of access into an EPU that is equipped with high-quality ultrasound have facilitated the early diagnosis of ectopic pregnancy. As ectopic pregnancy can be a life threatening condition, some form of intervention is usually undertaken. Although mortality rates are falling, ectopic pregnancy accounts for 80% of maternal deaths in the first trimester.[12]

The appearance of an ectopic pregnancy on TVUS is classically described as the 'bagel sign', which describes a hyperechoic ring around the gestation sac in the adnexal region (Figure 8.6). More often, however, an ectopic pregnancy is seen as a small, inconglomerate mass next to the ovary.

The use of TVUS has substantially increased the possibility of demonstrating an early ectopic pregnancy before major complications occur. The availability of TVUS and the facility to perform rapid ßhCG level analysis has significantly reduced the number of laparoscopies that are performed to exclude ectopic pregnancy. A gestational sac as small as 5 mm in diameter and a complex adnexal mass as small as 10 mm in diameter can be seen with TVUS. If the woman is compliant and the ectopic pregnancy is small, with no cardiac activity (the woman's liver function must be normal), methotrexate can be given as a single intramuscular dose titrated to the woman's height and weight (50 mg/m^2). Close

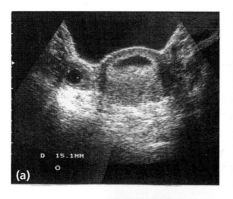
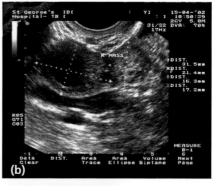

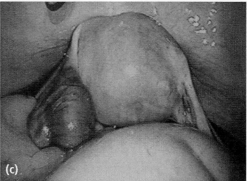

Figure 8.6 Ectopic pregnancy at 6 weeks' amenorrhoea seen **(a–b)** on transvaginal ultrasound scan and **(c)** at laparoscopy

ßhCG monitoring is then mandatory. Medical treatment using methotrexate is carried out in selected cases with close surveillance of ßhCG levels at day 4 and day 7, to confirm a downward trend, and follow-up is continued until levels have dropped below 10 iu/l. It is evident from the literature that single dose regimens can be used with confidence only when women present with low ßhCG levels. Many studies quote that between 2000 iu/l and 4000 iu/l give acceptable success rates (up to 92%).[13] There is an important role for EPUs in the ongoing care and support of women who are undergoing this method of management, for which 24 hour access is essential.

The evidence suggests that laparoscopic surgery improves patient morbidity and improves long-term reproductive outcomes.[14,15] This procedure also has the advantage of shortened hospital stay (1.3 days) and convalescence (2.4 weeks) compared with laparotomy, for which the respective figures are 3.1 days and 4.6 weeks.[11]

Expectant management is also used for women with ectopic pregnancy but the unpredictability and longevity of this method can increase anxiety levels for both patient and healthcare professional. A unit with 24 hour access, accurate ßhCG level estimation and high-resolution scanning facilities may meet the needs of these women. Initial serum ßhCG level appears to be the best predictor of outcome, with expectant management being successful in 96% of cases where the ßhCG level was initially less than 175 iu/l.[16]

There are units that use serum progesterone level as a clinical indicator for prediction of the viability of the pregnancy when attempting to refine the selection criteria for the use of expectant management. Elson *et al.*[16] state that in addition to clinical presentation and ßhCG level, 30% of ectopic pregnancies in women with a serum progesterone level of less than 10 nmol/l will resolve spontaneously, whereas in those with a serum progesterone level of more than 50 nmol/l the chance of resolution is slim. The use of this type of surveillance and decision-making requires senior, experienced health professionals and may not be practical in all situations.

Anti-immunoglobulin D

Women who are rhesus D negative should receive anti-immunoglobulin D if they have an ectopic pregnancy, are at more than 12 weeks' gestation with bleeding, have a surgical intervention or medical management for miscarriage, or if the miscarriage is accompanied by severe pain and heavy bleeding.[11]

Psychological aspects of early pregnancy loss

Support services and counselling should be identified to couples and should be available within the EPU. The EPU staff, although unable to provide all aspects of this important part of follow-up care, should be able to support the woman and her partner by giving information and contact numbers for available counselling and support networks.

Supporting literature

All aspects of management should be supported with up-to-date, evidence-based, written information. Included in this literature should be contact numbers for the EPU, local and national support networks, and internet addresses for recommended websites.

Emergency gynaecology

Many of the women who attend as gynaecological emergencies require the same one-stop service as women attending the EPU (Boxes 8.1 and 8.2). The majority of women can be managed in the ambulatory care environment and very few women require admission to hospital as inpatients. The criteria for hospital admission should be any condition that cannot be managed at home. This may

> **Box 8.3** Causes of acute pelvic pain that are not related to pregnancy
>
> - Pelvic inflammatory disease
> - Cyst accident (rupture or haemorrhage)
> - Adnexal torsion
> - Appendicitis
> - Fibroid degeneration
> - Others, e.g. constipation and urinary tract infection.

include high pyrexia, the need for opiate pain relief, intravenous antibiotics or further investigations that are only possible within a hospital environment.

The main indication for referral to the EGU is pelvic pain (Box 8.3). Transvaginal ultrasound scan is an effective means of detecting the cause of pelvic pain and is therefore an integral part of the one-stop service. This procedure is discussed in detail in Chapter 9.

Monitoring, audit and evaluation

Clinical effectiveness demands that the following questions be asked:

- What should be happening?
- What is happening?
- What changes are needed?

Data collection should reflect the requirements of ongoing audit of the service, particularly against national and local guidelines. Clinical audit is becoming one of the most vigorous methods for enabling clinical practice to be appraised against an evidence base, which is incorporated into guidelines. Government initiatives, including 'A First Class Service: Quality in the New NHS'[6] and the NHS Plan[3] have renewed the drive for audit through the introduction of clinical governance. This impetus has been supported by The National Institute for Health and Clinical Excellence,[2] which identified that clinical audit should be at the core of a system of local monitoring of performance and should be compulsory. The reasons given for absence of audit are usually lack of time and inexperience of personnel. It is essential, therefore, that the data are collected as part of the day-to-day statistic collection via a user-friendly database.

Conclusion

EPUs and EGUs are excellent examples of ambulatory gynaecology services where a one-stop management philosophy has been combined with minimal access daycase surgery to shorten the care pathway and avoid inpatient hospital admissions.

References

1. Bigrigg MA, Read MD. Management of women referred to early pregnancy assessment unit: care and cost effectiveness. *BMJ* 1991;302:577–9.
2. Department of Health, Department for Education and Skills. *National Service Framework for children, young people and maternity services*. London: The Stationery Office; 2004.
3. Department of Health. *The NHS Plan. A plan for investment, a plan for reform*. London: The Stationery Office; 2000.
4. Department of Health. *Better prevention, better services, better sexual health – The national strategy for sexual health and HIV*. London: The Stationery Office; 2001.
5. Royal College of Radiologists, Royal College of Obstetricians and Gynaecologists. *Guidance on ultrasound procedures in early pregnancy*. London: RCR and RCOG; 1995.
6. Department of Health. *A first class service: quality in the NHS*. London: The Stationery Office; 1998.
7. Blohm F, Hahlin M, Nielson S, Milsom I. Fertility after a randomised trial of spontaneous abortion managed by surgical evacuation or expectant treatment. *Lancet* 1997;349:995.
8. Nielsen S, Hahlin M, Platz-Christensen J. Randomised trial comparing expectant with medical management for first trimester miscarriages. *Br J Obstet Gynaecol* 1999;106:804–7.
9. Creinin MD, Moyer R, Guido R. Misoprostol for medical evacuation of early pregnancy failure. *Obstet Gynecol* 1997;89:768–72.
10. Zalanyi S. Vaginal misoprostol alone is effective in the treatment of missed abortion. *Br J Obstet Gynaecol* 1998;105:1026–8.
11. Royal College of Obstetricians and Gynaecologists. *The Management of Early Pregnancy Loss*. Clinical Guideline No. 25. London: RCOG; 2006.
12. Royal College of Obstetricians and Gynaecologists. *Why Mothers Die. The Fifth Report of the Confidential Enquiries into Maternal Deaths in the United Kingdom 1997–1999*. London: RCOG; 2001.
13. Tawfiq A, Agameya AF, Claman P. Predictors of treatment failure for ectopic pregnancy treated with single-dose methotrexate. *Fertil Steril* 2000;74:877–80.
14. Vermesh M, Silva PD, Rosen GF, Stein AL, Fossum GT, Sauer MV. Management of unruptured ectopic gestation by linear salpingostomy: a prospective, randomized clinical trial of laparoscopy versus laparotomy. *Obstet Gynecol* 1989;73:400–4.
15. Lundorff P, Thorburn J, Hahlin M, Kallfelt B, Lindblom B. Laparoscopic surgery in ectopic pregnancy. A randomized trial versus laparotomy. *Acta Obstet Gynecol Scand* 1991;70:343–8.
16. Elson J, Tailor A, Banergee S, Salim R, Hillaby K, Jurkovic D. Expectant management of tubal ectopic pregnancy: prediction of successful outcome using decision tree analysis. *Ultrasound Obstet Gynecol* 2004;23:552–6.

9

Pelvic ultrasound and interventional radiology

Woodruff Walker, Zara Haider and Tom Bourne

Introduction

Pelvic ultrasound scanning has a pivotal role in the provision of one-stop gynae-cology services. It is particularly important for abnormal uterine bleeding (Chapter 4), infertility (Chapter 7) and early pregnancy complications (Chapter 8). It is also the primary diagnostic tool for the investigation of acute pelvic pain in the emergency gynaecology unit.[1]

Transvaginal ultrasound scan

A natural extension of the gynaecological examination, a transvaginal ultra-sound scan (TVUS) should be used to confirm or exclude a diagnosis that is sus-pected on the basis of clinical findings. It is one of the least invasive diagnostic tools available. The transvaginal probe (5–7.5 MHz) produces a high-resolution image of the pelvic organs, providing reliable, reproducible information without the need for a full bladder.

TVUS has had a major impact on gynaecological practice. It is the investiga-tive tool of choice for triaging women with pelvic pain into appropriate treatment protocols, thus enabling the clinician to avoid surgery in some cases and select the best surgical approach in others. With the use of TVUS, common gynaecolog-ical pathology of the pelvic organs may be diagnosed with confidence. In the presence of a negative pregnancy test and a normal pelvic examination, a normal ultrasound scan gives reassurance that the risk of notable pelvic pathology is small.

Provision of a TVUS facility as part of an outpatient or emergency assessment makes sense for both doctor and patient. The doctor can relate their scan findings directly to the history and examination that preceded the scan. For the woman it means a one-stop service rather than several visits for initial consultation, the scan and for any subsequent tests indicated by the scan.

Causes of acute pelvic pain

Pelvic pain may be categorised as acute or chronic. No accurate definition of acute pelvic pain exists. Chronic pelvic pain is generally used to describe pain

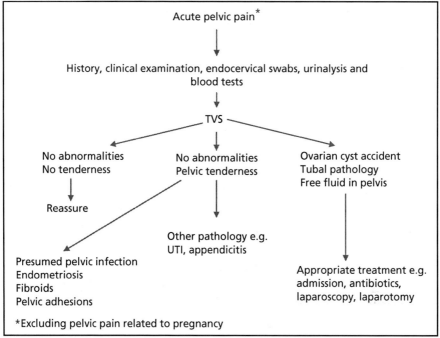

Figure 9.1 Management of acute pelvic pain

that has existed for more than 6 months. Acute pelvic pain is particularly suited to assessment by TVUS at the time of presentation in an emergency gynaecology unit. The pathway for assessment, investigation and diagnosis of acute pelvic pain (in nonpregnant women) is set out in a flow diagram (Figure 9.1).

Pelvic inflammatory disease

Sexually active young women between the ages of 16 and 25 years may present with deep dyspareunia and nonspecific pelvic pain rather than the vaginal discharge, severe pelvic pain, pyrexia and raised white cell count typically associated with pelvic inflammatory disease. The pelvic organs may all be tender on contact with the transvaginal probe because the ascending infection causes myometritis, endometritis, salpingitis and oophoritis. Fluid may be seen within the endometrial cavity and the endometrial shadow becomes less distinct than normal. The fallopian tubes are not routinely seen on greyscale ultrasound; however, inflammation leads to collection of fluid in the tube (Figure 9.2) as well as thickening of the walls. The tube is then seen as a cystic, sausage-shaped structure with swollen mucosal folds protruding into its lumen (cog-wheel effect). A tuboovarian abscess may be unilocular or multilocular, it may look solid and it may contain homogeneously echogenic material corresponding to pus (resembling an endometrioma on scan appearance).

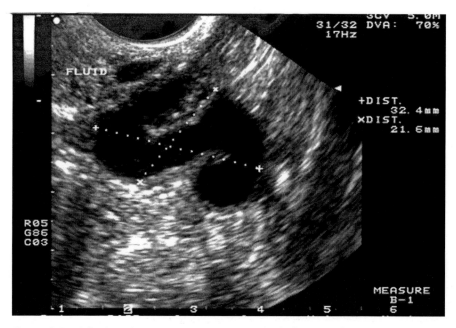

Figure 9.2   A hydrosalpynx seen on a transvaginal ultrasound scan

If the diagnosis of pelvic inflammatory disease is made on the basis of history, examination and scan appearance, unnecessary laparoscopy can be avoided. Prompt diagnosis and treatment with appropriate antibiotics reduces the incidence of tubal factor infertility and the subsequent risk of ectopic pregnancy.

Ovarian cyst accident

Ovarian cysts are a common incidental finding on a scan. If a woman with acute pelvic pain is found to have a cyst it may not necessarily be contributing to her pain. 7% of premenopausal women have cysts larger than 25 mm found on scan.[2] If pain is provoked by pushing on the cyst with the ultrasound probe, there may be a causative relationship.

Haemorrhagic corpus luteum is a common cause of acute pelvic pain in women of reproductive age (Figure 9.3). On TVUS, blood clots or a characteristic appearance similar to a spider's web may be seen within the cyst cavity. When Doppler flow is applied, a highly vascular flow is usually seen. Even a seemingly large corpus luteal cyst will usually disappear spontaneously.

All too often, unnecessary surgery is performed to remove the cyst. This procedure may result in significant blood loss owing to the vascular nature of the cyst. The most appropriate management is usually conservative, with administration of analgesia if required. The woman should be offered a follow-up scan at 6 weeks after surgery, for reassurance.

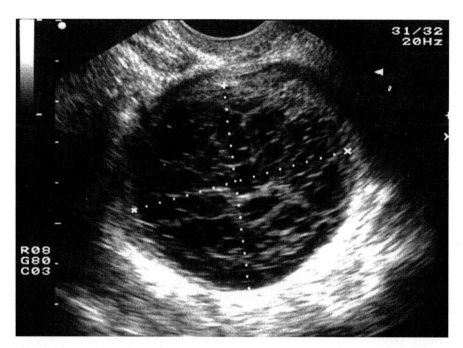

Figure 9.3 Haemorrhagic corpus luteum seen on a transvaginal ultrasound scan

Physiological rupture of an ovarian cyst is associated with mittelschmerz or mid-cycle pain. This pain is caused by irritation of the peritoneum by fluid or blood at the time of ovulation. A TVUS may demonstrate free fluid in the pouch of Douglas and a collapsed, flaccid cyst with an irregular wall. Surgical intervention should be avoided. Treated conservatively, the pain usually responds well to simple analgesia. The cyst should resolve spontaneously. A repeat scan should be performed after 6 weeks, for reassurance.

Adnexal torsion

Adnexal torsion usually occurs if the adnexa contain a lesion such as a hydrosalpinx or an ovarian cyst. It is difficult to diagnose adnexal torsion on ultrasound. The torsion leads to arterial and lymphatic occlusion. Congestion and oedema are classically followed with haemorrhage and infarction. On ovarian torsion, the affected ovary swells with oedema and appears large on the scan. If torsion occurs in an ovarian cyst or hydrosalpinx, the wall, mucosal folds and septa of the cyst appear swollen on ultrasound examination. If there is haemorrhagic infarction, blood (seen as echogenic fluid) may be present in the pouch of Douglas.

The use of Doppler imaging to look for absent or reduced vascular flow is not usually helpful because persistent arterial flow is compatible with less complete stages of torsion. A suspicion of torsion requires prompt surgical intervention.

Without intervention, the acute pain usually subsides owing to tissue death; by the time the pain has subsided, intervention with a view to preserving ovarian function is futile.

Fibroid degeneration

Fibroids themselves do not cause pain. Acute pain from fibroids is a result of degeneration or haemorrhage within the fibroid and, occasionally, torsion of a pedunculated fibroid. Ultrasound examination shows an increased size of the fibroid or uterus compared with previous examinations, cystic change within the fibroid, or both. Localised tenderness with use of the probe is strong evidence that the fibroid is the source of pain. A degenerating fibroid does not normally require surgical intervention. Often strong analgesia is required and the woman may need admission for symptom relief.

Interventional radiology in ambulatory gynaecology

Interventional radiology developed rapidly as a practice in the late 1960s and the 1970s. It became established particularly in general surgery, urology, vascular surgery and neurology with the increasing use of angioplasty balloons, stents and percutaneous drainage of abscesses and collections, and diagnostically through ultrasonography and computed tomography guided biopsies. Although the use of interventional radiology by gynaecologists has been delayed, angiographic embolisation has now become accepted as the treatment of choice for potentially life-threatening obstetric and gynaecological haemorrhage. Its effectiveness in these situations is now undisputed. Selected interventional radiological techniques are possible in gynaecological practice, and such procedures can be carried out in the outpatient setting, with minimal morbidity and complication rates. Fibroid embolisation is a minimal access technique that requires a short postoperative stay in hospital.

Ultrasound guided ovarian cyst aspiration

In the early 1980s, benign ovarian cysts were aspirated ultrasonically via a speculum placed in the vagina and under transvesical and transabdominal ultrasound guidance.[3] With improvements in transvaginal scanners it became possible to aspirate ovarian cysts transvaginally.

The technique is simple. Intravenous antibiotics are administered to cover the procedure, a transvaginal ultrasound probe with a biopsy guide (Figure 9.4) attached is placed in the vagina and the ovarian lesion is targeted. Under ultrasound control, a needle is then passed through the transvaginal probe and fluid from the cyst or collection is aspirated. The size of the needle is adjusted according to the predicted viscosity of the fluid. When endometriomas are being aspirated, a large-bore 14 or 16 gauge needle should be used. When serous-type fluid

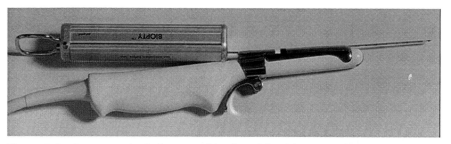

Figure 9.4   A transvaginal ultrasound probe with a biopsy guide

is being aspirated, an 18 or 20 gauge needle will suffice. If the ovarian cyst is easily accessible and thin-walled, it may not be necessary to administer intravenous sedation to cover the procedure. In the case of endometriomas or in more complex cases, however, intravenous sedation should be administered. A combination of midazolam (Hypnovel®, Roche, Welwyn Garden City, Herts), fentanyl and metoclopramide (Maxolon®, Shire, Basingstoke, Hants) titrated in small doses is usually sufficient.

The role of TVUS in the differential diagnosis of ovarian cysts prior to laparoscopic surgery has been described extensively.[4] The same preoperative diagnostic rules apply to cyst aspiration, which is another form of minimal access surgery, because the positive predicted value of ultrasound scanning for ovarian cysts is high.[5-7] It is important, however, that the cysts are unilocular and thin-walled if the technique is going to be successful and safe. Subtle, superficial, internal mural nodules or small papillary excrescences should be meticulously searched for because these features may indicate a malignant lesion, in particular a borderline tumour. With careful attention to ultrasound surveillance, cyst aspiration can be performed safely in both premenopausal and postmenopausal women.[8,9] In one-third to one-half of cases cyst aspiration will constitute definitive therapy. In other cases cysts will recur but may be followed up, depending on their rate of growth. Unfortunately, cytology alone is not sufficiently accurate to exclude malignancy.[10-12] Complex cysts seen on TVUS should not be managed by transvaginal aspiration because of the risk of malignancy.

Haemorrhagic cysts that do not resolve spontaneously or those that are symptomatic may be aspirated, usually via an 18 or 20 gauge needle, resulting in complete relief of symptoms.

Cyst aspiration in pregnant women is also feasible, and this technique is useful for functional cysts that become large and symptomatic.[3] By aspiration of the cyst, the possibility of rupture or torsion can be reduced. Cysts that persist into later pregnancy are more likely to be serous or mucinous cysts and may be malignant. In some cases it may, however, be useful to aspirate the cyst and to remove it postpartum. Such treatment may be warranted after careful assessment because surgical treatment for cysts in pregnancy is not without risk, with reported miscarriage rates between 2% and 35%.[13]

Transvaginal core biopsy of gynaecological lesions

A trial of fibroid embolisation has been carried out at the Royal Surrey County Hospital.[14] In a number of cases transvaginal guided core biopsy was found to be useful to assist the preoperative diagnosis. It was particularly useful when there was doubt about the diagnosis of adenomyoma versus fibroids or in cases where it was necessary to confirm a diagnosis of adenomyosis by magnetic resonance imaging. Transvaginal guided core biopsy also helps with the identification of a parauterine mass if there is uncertainty about whether it is an ovarian fibrothecoma or a pedunculated fibroid, or if there has been rapid growth of a fibroid with the possibility of the lesion being a sarcoma.[14] The technique is simple but it should be used with intravenous sedation, as described above. A 16 or 18 gauge core biopsy needle, mounted on a biopsy gun (Figure 9.4), is introduced through the vagina to the targeted area of the uterus via the myometrium (Figure 9.5).

If it is necessary to confirm a diagnosis of adenomyosis, it is important that the endometrium is avoided. Several cores of myometrium should be obtained and submitted for histological diagnosis. The accuracy of the technique is high even in adenomyosis where, of nine women subsequently operated on, the correct diagnosis of adenomyosis was made in eight of the women. In one woman adenomyosis was diagnosed but the myometrium was considered normal on histological assessment.[14]

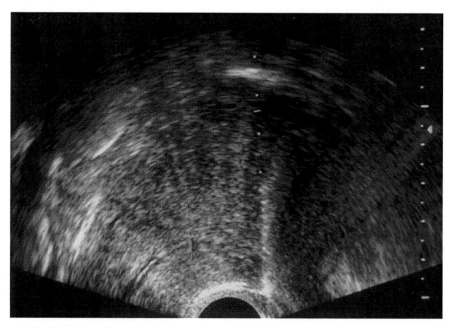

Figure 9.5 A biopsy gun is introduced through the vagina to the targeted area of the uterus via the myometrium (dotted line), as seen on transvaginal ultrasound scan

Ovarian cyst aspiration and transvaginal core biopsy are simple techniques that can be used in the office setting and may avoid the need for surgery or increase preoperative or interventional diagnostic confidence.

Selective salpingography and fallopian tube catheterisation and tuboplasty

Selective salpingography and fallopian tube catheterisation, sometimes combined with balloon dilatation of fallopian tubes, has been used in the diagnosis and treatment of infertility. Although this procedure has a high success rate in selected women it still appears under-used in obstetric and gynaecological practice in the UK. A reason for this under-use may be that the technique was adopted mainly by gynaecologists who were driven by pressure from firms selling equipment for selective salpingography. Although the procedure may sometimes be easy, it can prove technically difficult, requiring a skilled interventional radiologist and the use of microcatheters and microwires and, in some cases, small balloons. In order to perform selective salpingography the woman should be sedated as described above. After insertion of a speculum, the cervix is grasped using volsellum forceps and, particularly if a difficult procedure is anticipated, a bilateral paracervical block, using lignocaine, is administered. An introduction catheter fitted with a uterine balloon is then placed in the uterus and a hysterosalpingogram is performed, with a good cervical seal. When the proximal tubal occlusion is identified a shaped catheter is then passed through the introduction catheter and very carefully placed at the uterine cornu. It is at this point that skilled interventional techniques are necessary in order to pass a fine microcatheter and guidewire through the proximal occlusion and not perforate the fallopian tube (Figure 9.6).

Interventional radiologists are used to using hydrophilic microcatheters and microwires and these are often necessary for the catheterisation. Interventional radiologists successfully catheterise proximally occluded fallopian tubes in 71–92% of cases and pregnancy rates after the procedure are variable but with an average rate of 30%.[15] Recanalisation is also possible in women who have had

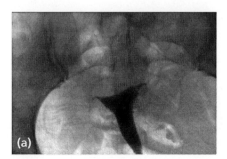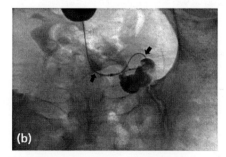

Figure 9.6 **(a)** Initial hysterosalpingography showing bilateral cornual blocks and **(b)** selective recanalisation of the left fallopian tube with microcatheter (arrow on left) and guidewire (arrow on right), with free spill at the end of the procedure

occlusion after surgical anastomosis or reversal of tubal ligation. In addition, recanalisation may be successful in women with occlusion related to salpingitis isthmica nodosa but the procedure is technically more difficult in such circumstances.[16] Although recanalisation has a high success rate, approximately 38% of tubes reblock after 6–12 months. In these patients repeated recanalisation is usually successful.[15,17]

Fibroid embolisation

Background

The first case of uterine artery embolisation for fibroids was performed by a neuroradiologist, Jean-Jacques Merland, in Paris in 1974. In 1996, a trial of fibroid embolisation was commenced at the Royal Surrey County Hospital, Guildford, and to date over 1,300 women have been treated,[17] with a median follow-up period of 16.7 months.[18] Embolisation achieved an average shrinkage of more than 67% and the success rate in terms of symptom relief exceeded 85%. In subsequent papers[19,20] the authors analysed effectiveness in relation to the types of fibroids embolised and pregnancy rates. Fibroid embolisation was effective for small, large, single or multiple fibroids and a series of 26 full-term pregnancies occurred following uterine artery embolisation[20] (Figure 9.7).

Although uterine artery embolisation can be technically difficult, in most cases an interventional radiologist who is trained in the technique can perform it rapidly (usually in less than 1 hour) and without difficulty. The procedure is not amenable to the outpatient setting and it does need to be performed in an interventional vascular suite, but it is a minimal access technique.

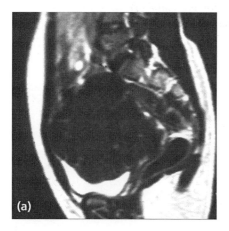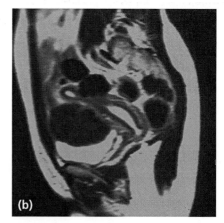

Figure 9.7 **(a)** A large fibroid mass before embolisation and **(b)** shrinkage of fibroids and some cavity compression followed by successful pregnancy after embolisation, both seen on magnetic resonance imaging (sagittal T2-weighted images)

The procedure

Under intravenous sedation and antibiotic cover, a small catheter is placed in the femoral artery. Under X-ray television control and using combinations of stand-ard catheters and guidewires, a microcatheter is manipulated into the uterine artery and placed approximately one-half to two-thirds of the way along the vis-ualised length of the artery. In most cases polyvinyl alcohol particles, 355–500 μm in diameter and diluted appropriately, are injected through the catheter until the branches of the uterine artery are occluded (Figure 9.8).

In a small number of women, the desired result can be obtained by embolisa-tion of only one vessel, if the other uterine artery clearly supplies the normal uterus. If there is any doubt concerning the efficacy of the procedure – that is, whether complete fibroid infarction has been obtained – a gadolinium enhanced dynamic magnetic resonance imaging scan (Figure 9.9) can be used to identify any residual vascular perfusion of the fibroid or fibroids.

Following this procedure the woman suffers a variable degree of pain, which may in some cases be severe. We treat this pain by giving the woman a patient-controlled morphine pump and anti-inflammatory drugs. Following the proce-dure the woman is discharged the following day and requires 1–2 weeks of convalescence.

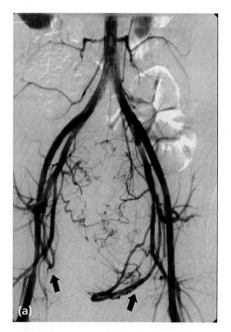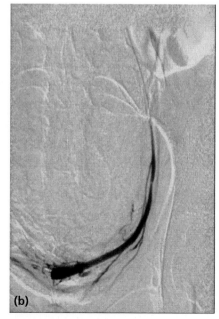

Figure 9.8 Flush arteriogram showing **(a)** dilated uterine arteries (arrows) and hypervascular fibroid mass and **(b)** left uterine artery following embolisation by polyvinyl alcohol particles

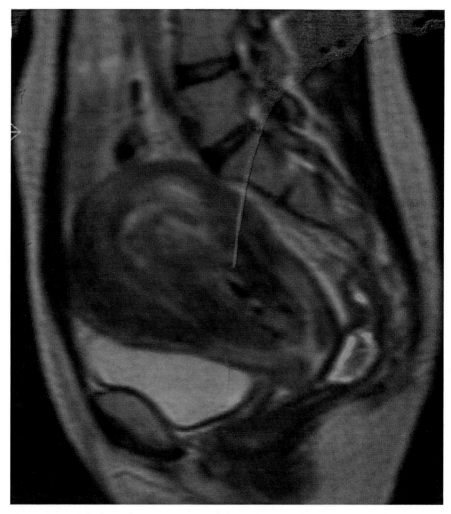

Figure 9.9 Infarcted fibroids and normal perfusion of the uterus seen on a post-gadolinium magnetic resonance imaging scan

Complications

Ovarian failure has been a feared complication of uterine artery embolisation but in fact this problem is rare and it has an incidence of less than 1% in patients under the age of 45 years.[20,21] Vaginal discharge can be a problem after embolisation[20] but it is usually self-limited. If discharge is persistent it can usually be cured by a hysteroscopic resection.[20] Infection may, in rare instances, require a hysterectomy.

Women may either pass their fibroids spontaneously or require hysteroscopic removal (Figure 9.10). We have had many cases of large submucous fibroids, for which myomectomy would have been an extremely difficult procedure, that have

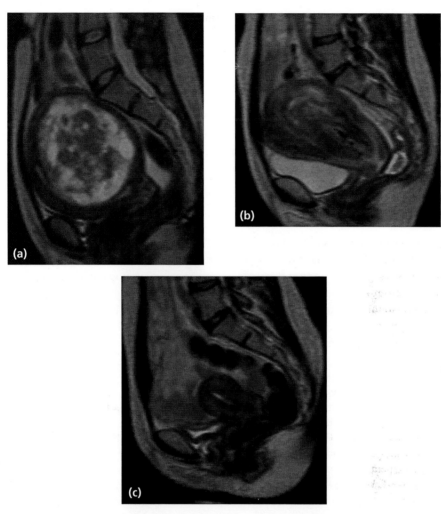

Figure 9.10 T2-weighted sagittal magnetic resonance images showing **(a)** a large submucous fibroid, **(b)** an infarcted, crenated fibroid in the uterine lumen with early dilatation of the endocervical canal and **(c)** normal uterus seen after a hysteroscopic resection

culminated in a normal uterus following embolisation and subsequent hysteroscopic resection. Hysteroscopic resection of an infarcted, crenated, intracavitary fibroid is substantially easier than attempted hysteroscopic resection of a large hypervascular fibroid.

Recent advances

A combined procedure has been developed in which embolisation followed by myomectomy (laparoscopic or open) are carried out consecutively, on the same day. This procedure is usually performed in two categories of women who wish to preserve their fertility. The first is women with large (more than 25 cm in diameter), numerous and complex fibroid masses in which neither procedure would be likely to succeed alone. Embolisation produces a virtually bloodless field for the gynaecologist and any fibroids left behind will be killed by the embolisation. The second category is women who have masses that are smaller but that comprise a combination of interstitial and submucous fibroids, as well as a notable pedunculated fibroid or fibroids. Pedunculated fibroids do not respond well to embolisation but can easily be removed surgically. Also, pedunculated fibroids that are larger than would normally be attempted laparascopically can be removed via the laparoscope because of the relatively bloodless field.

Conclusion

Pelvic ultrasound scanning plays a pivotal role in the provision of one-stop gynaecology services. This technique is particularly important for the investigation of acute pelvic pain in the emergency gynaecology unit where it can prevent women from undergoing a laparoscopy under general anaesthesia. Advances in interventional radiology have resulted in techniques that can be applied to women with gynaecological pathology and these procedures provide outpatient-based alternatives to minimal access or conventional surgery.

References

1. Okaro E, Condous G, Bourne T. The use of ultrasound in the management of gynaecological conditions. In: Studd J, editor. *Progress in Obstetrics and Gynaecology,* vol 15. Edinburgh: Churchill Livingstone; 2003. p. 273–97.
2. Okaro E, Condous G, Khalid A, Timmerman D, Wang X, Van Huffel S, *et al.* Does a normal scan exclude the presence of significant pathology in women with chronic pelvic pain. *Ultrasound Med Biol* 2003;29 Suppl 1:25.
3. Khaw KT, Walker WJ. Ultrasound guided fine needle aspiration of ovarian cysts: diagnosis and treatment in pregnant and non-pregnant women. *Clin Radiol* 1990;41:105–8.
4. De Crespigny L. Laparoscopic ovarian surgery: Preoperative diagnosis and imaging. In: Sutton C, Diamond MP, editors. *Endoscopic Surgery for Gynaecologists.* 2nd ed. London: WB Saunders; 1998. p 201–11.
5. Granberg S, Crona N, Enk L, Hammarberg K, Wikland M. Ultrasound-guided puncture of cystic tumors in the lower pelvis of young women. *J Clin Ultrasound* 1989;17:107–11.
6. Granberg S, Nostrom A, Wikland M. Tumors in the lower pelvis as imaged by vaginal sonography. *Gynecol Oncol* 1990;37:224–9.
7. Moyle JW, Rochester D, Sider L, Shrock K, Krause P. Sonography of ovarian tumors: predictability of tumor type. *AJR Am J Roentgenol* 1983;141:985–91.
8. Troiano RN, Taylor KJ. Sonographically guided therapeutic aspiration of benign-appearing ovarian cysts and endometriomas. *AJR Am J Roentgenol* 1998;171:1601–5.

9. Caspi B, Goldchmit R, Zalel Y, Appelman Z, Insler V. Sonographically guided aspiration of ovarian cyst with simple appearance. *J Ultrasound Med* 1996;15:297–300.

10. Dordoni D, Zaglio S, Zucca S, Favalli G. The role of sonographically guided aspiration in the clinical management of ovarian cysts. *J Ultrasound Med* 1993;12:27–31.

11. Granberg S, Wickland M, Jansson I. Macroscopic characterization of ovarian tumors and the relation to the histological diagnosis: criteria to be used for ultrasound evaluation. *Gynecol Oncol* 1989;35:139–44.

12. Granberg S, Wikland M. Ultrasound in the diagnosis and treatment of ovarian cystic tumours. *Hum Reprod* 1991;6:177–85.

13. Buttery BW, Beischer NA, Fortune DW, Macafee CA. Ovarian tumours in pregnancy. *Med J Aust* 1973;1:345–9.

14. Walker WJ, Jones K. Transvaginal ultrasound guided biopsies in the diagnosis of pelvic lesions. *Minim Invasive Ther Allied Technol* 2003;12:241–4.

15. Thurmond AS, Machan LS, Maubon AJ, Rouanet JP, Hovsepian DM, Van Moore A, *et al.* A review of selective salpingography and fallopian tube catherization. *Radiographics* 2000;20:1759–68.

16. Thurmond AS, Brandt KR, Gorrill MJ. Tubal obstruction after ligation reversal surgery: results of catheter recanalization. *Radiology* 1999;210:747–50.

17. Dover RW, Sutton CJG, Walker WJ. Arterial embolisation for uterine fibroids. The results of the largest UK series. *BJOG* 1998;105(Supplement 17):52.

18. Walker WJ, Pelage JP. Uterine artery embolisation for symptomatic fibroids: clinical results in 400 women with imaging follow up. *BJOG* 2002;109:1262–72.

19. Watson GM, Walker WJ. Uterine artery embolisation for the treatment of symptomatic fibroids in 114 women: reduction in size of the fibroids and women's views of the success of the treatment. *BJOG* 2002;109:129–35.

20. Goodwin SC, Bonilla SM, Sacks D, Reed RA, Spies JB, Landow WJ, *et al.* Reporting standards for uterine artery embolization for the treatment of uterine leiomyomata. *J Vasc Interv Radiol* 2001;12:1011–20.

21. Chrisman HB, Saker MB, Ryu RK, Nemcek AA Jr, Gerbie MV, Milad MP, *et al.* The impact of uterine fibroid embolization on resumption of menses and ovarian function. *J Vasc Interv Radiol* 2000;11:699–703.

Index